A PEBBLE IN MY SHOE

CHRIS MAWSON

First edition A pebble in my shoe © **Copyright 2017 Chris Mawson**

Illustration © **Copyright 2017 by Chris Mawson**

All rights reserved. No part of this publication may be reproduced, Stored in a retrieval system (other than for the purposes of review) Without prior permission of the author/copyright holder.

ISBN: 978-1978387386

A catalogue record of this book is available from the National library of Australia.

Chris Mawson, A pebble in my shoe, first edition

Cover image by Chris Mawson © **Copyright 2017**

Cover design Chris Mawson © **Copyright 2017**

Edited and proof reading by Leeanne Hayes

This book is dedicated to my beautiful wife Sharon, without whom, these books would never have seen the light of day. Thank you for your love and support and kicking my arse in times of need.

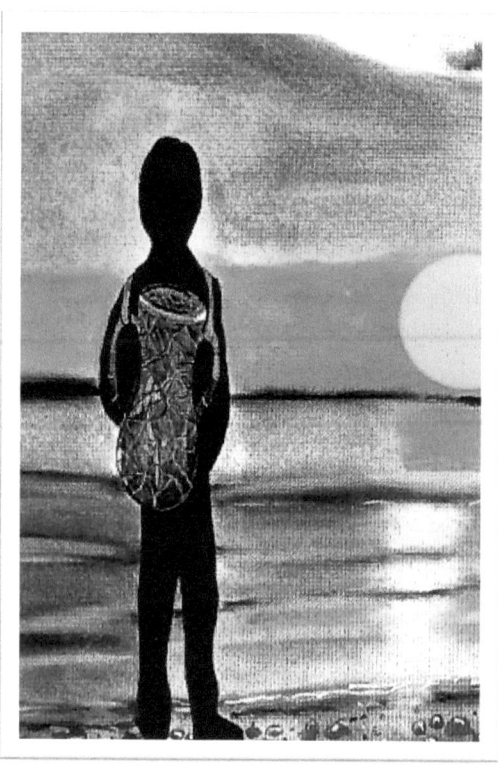

FOREWORD

As previously explored with powerful rawness and painful honesty in Chris's first book, 'Broken', the reader is made aware of the gravity of PTSD.

Chris is living proof that life is an ongoing journey and having suffered PTSD is only one part of that journey. Treatment, the support of a loving family and changes to how he chose to move forward, he now brings us his second book.

By writing these books, he brings hope to other PTSD sufferers as he speaks of dark times, through positive change and enjoying life. In the time I have known Chris, he has continued to work on his own personal growth and his confidence has flourished.

Linda Mouw

Credentialed Mental Health Nurse.

FOREWORD BY THE AUTHOR

My first book *'Broken'*, for many of you who read it, was a somewhat graphic and personal insight of my battle with PTSD within the ambulance service and my role as a paramedic.

The feedback I received after its publication was positively overwhelming. The main purpose of writing it was to encourage emergency service workers, who have suffered or are suffering with mental illness, as a direct result of the job they do, to come forward and hold up their hand and seek help.

Also, its aim was to gain awareness and prove through treatment and support, it is possible to overcome and live a near normal life.

Having been inundated with messages and kind words of thanks from paramedics, fire-fighters and police officers from around the world who are fighting their own battles, it confirms to me that PTSD is gradually becoming, if not already, a global epidemic.

Partners of those fighting have also reached out to me wanting to know the magic formula to overcome the darkest ebbs of the illness to help a wife, husband, mum or dad through the lengthy battle. There have been those who have realised from reading *'Broken'* that they now have a problem and it is time to tell someone at work or a family member. There is no magic formula to overcoming PTSD and each case is a personal, private battle with one's self. It's a long hard road without short cuts.

What worked for me may not work for someone else, but it is important to start somewhere. For me, my starting points were: -

Recognising I needed help and Accepting help.

These are the two hardest things to do - I will be the first to agree. Once you are over that hurdle then work can begin on the road to recovery with professional help and support.

The whole experience of writing **'Broken'** has humbled me to the core. It was written initially to help me through my darkest days and in the beginning, I was reluctant to share my personal and private thoughts to the world. I am thankful it has done some good and that individuals have taken pockets of my work away to help in their own quest for answers or indeed relate to the things I have experienced.

I do feel **'Broken'** on reflection seemed somewhat unfinished. Many wanted to know how I have "ended up" after such a lengthy battle...well I'm still here.... I "ended up" ... OK... and survived to tell the tale. But if truth be known, at the time of writing, I was in a deep, dark hole and it was close to being shelved!! I'm thankful I didn't and grateful that my wife Sharon encouraged me to push through. Those of you who know me or had been aware of my plight would probably understand.

It is now I feel ready to write a second book, '*A pebble in my shoe*'. This book is the conclusion to the battle I have endured over the last 3 years or more and a battle that is still ongoing. Once again it is open and frank. I truly wish that this too offers hope to those who are now hurting.

Best wishes – *CHRIS MAWSON*

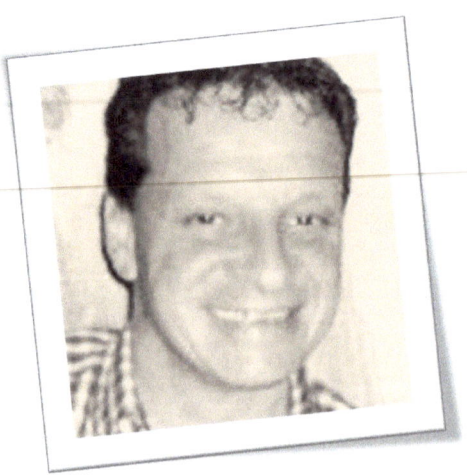

The idea of the jug used in *'BROKEN'* and *'A PEBBLE IN MY SHOE'.*

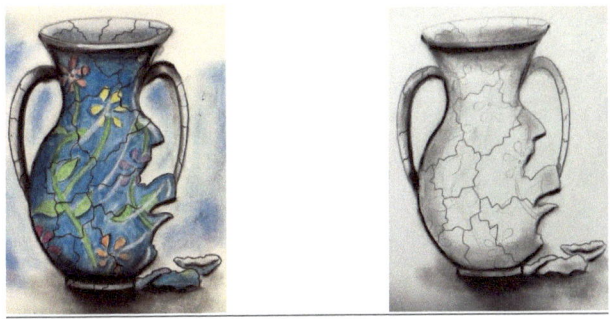

Many people have asked how the idea of the jug on the front cover in my previous book '***Broken***' and now carried through in this one came about.

The general idea came to my wife in a dream as she had dreamt about a broken jug, an analogy she felt best described my illness and '***Broken***' was initially penned with the title '***The broken jug***'. Her idea of a broken jug summed up in a nut shell, everything that PTSD and mental illness is.

Ironically only one week later and puzzled as to how the jug was to be illustrated in the way of colour, shape etc., we embarked on a day trip, exploring the smaller towns, south of Perth, Western Australia, ending up in a place called Donnybrook. A town that prides itself and famous for growing some of the best home-grown apples and fresh produce in Australia.

Even the street lamps fashioned as apples bow in acknowledgement to the towns pride of a product that has become a staple form of nourishment in our daily lives.

Whilst in search of a well-deserved lunch, we stumbled across an antique /gift shop with door open and the distinct aroma of incense seeping from within. Both being suckers for mooching around shops full of bygone objects we stepped inside. Within seconds of us entering, the puzzle was solved, for stood in front of us was a large vase/jug. The colours and shape of which are depicted on the front cover of both books.

There is now a subtle difference in how both jugs are represented on the cover of each book. There is naturally the obvious observation in that on the cover of 'Broken', pieces are missing from the jug and therefore scattered at its base. This in emphasis as to where we both sadly saw my mental state and life at that time... BROKEN.

Then comes the cover for this book which also depicts the jug being carried upon the back of a man stood by the shore at sunset. The jug is now complete in its form and the cracks of the jug sealed by gold and the sunset is acknowledgement that the sun is setting on a personal battle and making way for a new beginning. The symbol of the gold sealing the cracks of the jug is symbolised in an ancient Japanese tradition, known as Kintsugi. An analogy that is now kindred with the mental struggle bestowed on me in past years.

The broken jug has now been adopted as a background on posters at Australian mental health conferences and has been used at a paramedic symposium in Sydney (2016). Something I am extremely proud to be involved with. It seems the jug has in some way become a symbol of PTSD and mental illness.

It isn't the mountains ahead that wear you down.
It's the pebble inside your shoe–

                                      Mohammed Ali

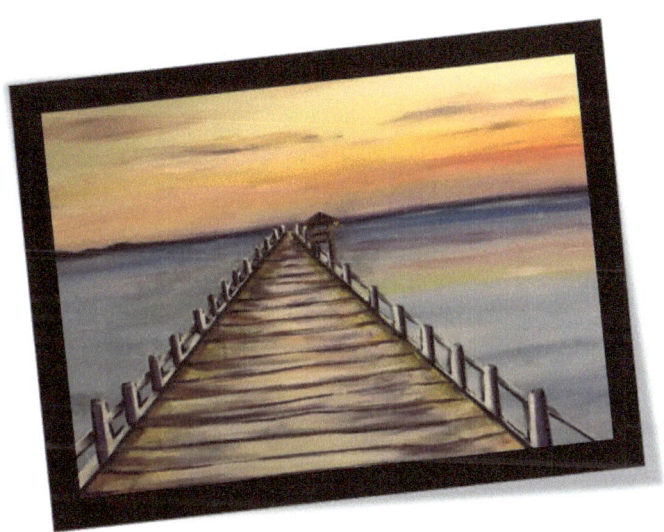

Chapter one

Frozen

I lay on my bed rigid, pale and shaking with waves of pain enveloping my body, mainly throat and stomach. Frozen to the spot, the room spins as I open my eyes to try and compensate for the post "rollercoaster ride" feeling that commands attention from my mind. I remember my therapy and all the tools I must use to combat the feelings and thoughts that naturally come into play. But it is hard work some days and today is no exception.

I inhale deep until it hurts and then exhale slowly, until every breath has left my body. I repeat several times, as the pain within me dissipates and I start to resemble a being of normal stature. It's funny how an ordinary shopping trip can dampen your day!

It's all about adaption to life again in my case. PTSD and the symptoms that accompany it, rears its ugly head frequently. How I deal with it is all in my hands.

There are certain parameters for me when shopping and crowds are one burden I must learn to cope with again. That is the biggest hindrance and defines a successful shopping experience or a "bugger it I'm out of here", experience.

The sounds that are normal to most in a shopping mall are the sounds that I must work on. If I generally recognise a sound, I'm not too bad unless someone is whistling or talking loudly on a phone. Even a loud bang makes the hairs on the back of my neck stand on end and rattles every nerve in my body.

If my mind can't make head nor tail of a sound, then that's when I become edgy and anxious. I know I must either walk away or fight the feelings that follow. I know it may seem petty to some, but this for many with PTSD or mental illness can be a big deal. It's that fight or flight syndrome which so often becomes more prevalent in daily life and becomes a constant battle of inner will.

When I was working as a paramedic, fight or flight was very much prevalent and magnified within the job I did. But decisions were so easy to make. There was no question that your mind was conditioned to making quick, calculated decisions because people's lives and wellbeing depended on that. Now it's a very different world and it takes time for my mind to compute and triage the good energy from the bad and what the mind perceives as safety or danger.

I was always told by my psychologist during my treatment; if I ever had this insecure feeling of edginess or hypervigilance to stop, look down at my body and quickly assess.

Was I bleeding?

Was I injured?

If the answer was no to both, then I was safe and ok. It then helps to put things in perspective and from there a conscious decision could be made. Using this method works most of the time, other times I would have gone beyond the point of no return. Fuel is thrown on the anxiety's fire and the beginnings of a panic attack would start to bubble.

My biggest pet hate is the self-serve check-out which I try to avoid at all cost. There is always that staff member that hovers around you, waiting to pounce on the basket you are just about to empty. You know they are behind you. You can feel their breath on the back of your neck as your self-scanning your goods. Then all hope of privacy has evaporated and personal space compromised.

This experience for me is magnified a hundred times as I know a sales assistant is behind me, but my brain tells me it's a mass murderer, with a twelve-inch machete. Then I become uneasy and agitated and I immediately slip into defensive mode. I will say nothing and stop what I am doing until they think something is wrong and ask if I need assistance or, look at me as if I'm deranged and walk away.

Generally, the latter happens, and all is good. On the way out, I just smile at the assistant and bid her good day. When she smiles back I am sure her thoughts are "what a weirdo!" as I clutch my carrier bags and head for glory. Or maybe it's just me, over analysing things, another problem that PTSD has.

Things that wouldn't have bothered me years ago when shopping, seem harder to deal with now and affect me more mentally. But my response has softened and as a cliché to the chapter title, I generally just "let it go".

Driving is another big issue for me and there are some days that I can manage and others when I would just have to give it a miss. I see the car these days as a four-wheeled monster. A David and Goliath type of thing and I think as I approach it, open the door, sit down and turn the key…… "will I conquer today?"

But there are days I need to take back up, in the form of my wife Sharon. It's not too bad if Sharon is in the car with me and there have been many occasions when I have had to pull over and let her take the wheel. If I pass an accident whilst driving that's when I start to feel anxious. Or I go into a transient focused state and drive faster. To the extent, I must be roused and told to slow down.

This can only be associated with the job I did, when seeing an accident and wanting to get to a scene, quickly. My mind goes into overdrive and for years trained to respond in such a manner. You could say it was a form of institutionalisation from serving as a Paramedic. That mind set is still there and is still hard to shake off.

The result of an episode like this generally ends in tremors, sweating, nausea, chest pain and sometimes remorseful emotion.... Oh, and a place in the passenger seat!

There have been times when driving, that Sharon has seen something that she knows will trigger me such as an accident, a passing emergency vehicle with flashing lights or even heavy traffic. She will start to talk about anything to avert my mind from being able to absorb and over analyse a situation. This is an attribute she has developed throughout my illness and understanding. It has been a total learning curve for her and something I am so grateful for. She is like my assistance wife, I swear every guy needs one!

But seriously speaking, being able to talk to her about my feelings has helped enormously, something I could never do previously. In the past talking about my feelings would trigger an argument and she would spend days walking on eggshells. I tended to nurture my thoughts and certain issues were buried as I struggled to come to terms with my demons. Sharon has learned to read a change in my demeanour or facial expression and intercept.

Each day bringing its challenges and some days more challenging than others. I never know how my day is going to play out until I am fully awake and can gauge my feelings. Some days are a total right off and I am unable to venture any further than the front door.

Daily tasks can be a chore and it sometimes takes effort to complete the simplest. Although I will say that cooking and ironing are still my favourite things to do at home and help to elevate the triggers that other tasks may bring.

There are many other things that I have had to learn to cope with all over again and my life has been changed in so many ways. I have adapted my daily regime in a structured manner and I must say I am much happier with myself and my outlook on life. It would have been so easy to lick my wounds and stay in bed day in day out, or fester feelings of being sorry for myself watching TV.

There are also times if someone is talking to me, I will be away with the fairies. I will sub consciously stare at the person, seemingly engaged in conversation with them, nodding periodically in acknowledgement to what they are saying. Then it turns to embarrassment when that same person is looking for a response and I ask them to repeat. I have no clue as to what the conversation was about.

I am there in the moment, but really, I'm on planet '*zip-a-dee-doo-dah*' – with Mr Bluebird on my shoulder. This is mainly due to brain overload as most days I'm still trying to digest what happened yesterday. The cogs are spinning in my mind, but I still can't find a place for yesterday's information.

I have now got to a stage where I can look in the mirror and see hope as opposed to the vile hate, I once had for the person looking back. No longer is that person a useless failure. No longer is that person someone I want to eradicate from life. There is now light at the end of the tunnel. The challenging work through therapy, perusing my hobbies of art, writing and music along with family support, has made me realise that there is something to live for once again. The fruits of the arduous work coupled with positivity have made me a stronger person. It has made Sharon and I a stronger couple.

My eating habits have changed vastly. As an Englishman born and bred on meat and two veg, the one thing I miss is my Sunday roast. No longer can I eat red meat.

Roast beef and a good old Yorkshire pudding with lashings of gravy are out. Red meat upsets my stomach now as it reminds me of trauma and my appetite has diminished with smaller portions. White meat, fish, salad and veggies are now the order of the day. Raw foods, salads and vegetables are now on the menu, with juicing now a given passion. Sharon calls it "happy food". I think she has a point!!

Many moons ago I would have laughed when she said that to me. I loved my big over faced feasts and she would be happy with a modest plate of fish and greens.

"But I'm from the north of England! That's how we eat", I would say.

Now I get it. A different mindset regarding nutritional intake is so very important in mental illness; along with exercise such as walking, cycling and swimming.

My personal view is if you feel good on the inside, you're sure to feel better on the outside. A common cliché, but so very true and has helped me enormously. It is mainly a case of motivation which so many find hard in mental illness, it is something I sympathise with.

Meditation is also common place in my life. I found it quite hard initially as having the skill to shut down the mind is not an easy task. It has been a case of trial and error, but I can compose myself enough to benefit. Negative thoughts generally turn to the positive and knowing that I am safe which helps me to relax.

The darker symptoms of PTSD are far and few between now, as far as thoughts go, but I occasionally still get suicidal feelings. Not to the extent I actively want to do anything, but it sometimes just comes to me as a passing suggestion. I would never act on those thoughts other than to tell Sharon. Something I could never do before. She can generally analyse quickly why I feel like that. We have a quick chat and that's it, all good.

Night time is generally a time when the bizarre and strange things happen. That's when the flash backs erratically come out to play. There are no warning signs and I never know when a dream will end in a gruesome night's sleep. The only thing I can do is limit the chance of allowing those dreams turning into something more sinister.

For instance, I avoid watching movies with extreme violence or horror. Certain news items I shy away from with upsetting content. Discussions with family in the evenings are generally kept light hearted and I treat evenings as a time to relax or wind down. Inevitably there are times when triggers are hard to avoid and unfortunately, they are carried to my slumber.

When I fail to protect my thoughts, there is generally one of two things that occur. The first being a simple nightmare which will incorporate flashbacks with generalised sleep talking or restlessness. Eventually surfacing at 4am for a cup of tea and a head scratch and back to bed. The talking is normally mumbled discussion between me or whoever, with sporadic shouting or mild grunting. This may last between thirty seconds and ten minutes, but I will have no recollection of anything I had been dreaming about.

The nightmares and dreams I do remember are inevitably to do with past jobs I had attended as a paramedic. It will never be the full scenario but more splinters of incidents. It may involve a nightmare where I am trapped in a burning car or building with no way out or the face of someone who is in deep distress. Someone who has been murdered, someone who has died at a scene I've attended. The face of a child I could not save or the last breath of a person as they slip away in front of my eyes. They and many more are constant visions that occupy my mind most nights. My mind is mostly a labyrinth of cogs that spin away carrying memories. Memories that I know will always stay with me, but to find a home in my mind for them is sometimes hard. I always wonder do they need a home in my mind? That's a tough call and some would think a selfish statement but certainly a debatable question.

If only it was as easy as putting them into a big box or an old tea chest and discarding them in a dark dusty room, until the end of time. Unfortunately, these sorts of memories have a way of escaping and no box now is strong enough to contain the energy they expel. The battle to eradicate these dreams is like sitting on top of the box and feeling the pounding on the lid as they try to escape. You fight and fight to keep them in there, but sometimes it becomes tiring and the mind becomes drained of energy.

Then you wake to start a new day and you feel as though you have never slept. That's why I understand it's easy for some people just to sleep the day away because in a world of PTSD there is no such thing as quality sleep.

Then life becomes a chore and there are no limits to irrationality and mood swings through lack of sleep. It can become a vicious cycle. Working hard to break the cycle can be achieved but certainly not easy. That's why I find meditation and exercise a fantastic release. Ongoing therapy also acts as a safety net and as

I have done over and over I am mostly able to toss my bad memories and dreams aside.

I also network my mind to compensate for negative thoughts with the use of art, music and writing. Some of my worst nights are also governed by the feeling that I have not achieved anything. So now I always make a concerted effort to accomplish something in my day, whether it be a painting, writing or a few household chores. The feeling of achievement makes for a goodnight sleep and a feeling of self-worth.

Another form of dreams or nightmares are the ones I act out. These dreams take the form of sleep walking. I had never been known to sleep walk. However, since being diagnosed with PTSD, I found out that this was what I was doing. I was in total disbelief and a little embarrassed. My wife Sharon would tell me the details the next morning after an event. It was only after some time that I asked her to video me as I wanted to see for myself how these episodes had played out.

The first time I viewed the footage I was astounded as to how disturbing my actions were. Generally, it would involve sitting up in bed first and talking in an incomprehensible tongue, mumbling and grunting like a wild caged animal.

Then stepping out of bed I would peak through the blinds draped at the window and I would become more animated and vocal. It was if I had seen something through the window in the front garden that had annoyed me, and I would start to shout at whoever or whatever was in my line of vision. Then begins the antics of opening and closing draws to find clothes to put on. I would don a baseball cap and sunglasses and walk around the room grunting periodically and shouting in frustration, looking like an E grade rapper void of rhyme or reason with the voice of an ape.

"Come back to bed Chris your safe", Sharon would say repeatedly, being careful not to wake or startle me.

She would repeat this until eventually I was back in bed. An average episode lasting up to 1 hour. I must say she had the patience of a saint and proved great testimony to her strength and belief in me.

One night I tried to put on Sharon's sarong thinking they were a pair of trousers. Have you any idea how hard these bloody things are to put on? It took me a good ten minutes of stumbling and fumbling until eventually I gave up much to my anger and frustration!

Other nights I would source tubes of creams from cupboards in the bathroom or bedroom and physically eat them. Sun tan lotion, hand cream, I wasn't really fussed. Then Sharon would grab whatever substance I was consuming from my hand and endeavour to pluck it from my mouth whilst I was still actively walking.

But I guess the episode I can now look back and laugh at was the time I rose, shouting and stumbling around the bedroom with a pillow firmly anchored on my head and then reaching for a bottle of rescue remedy. I downed the whole bottle in one!!

"Come back to bed, you are definitely safe now Chris", Sharon said with tears of laughter running down her face.

These episodes would confirm that my subconscious was acting out past events or jobs in a passively weird way. Often the next day I would feel as though I had not slept at all, as with other nightmares I experienced. I was never able to open a door thankfully. Who knows what would have happened if I'd got hold of the car keys!

Sharon's biggest fear was that I would become physically violent towards her but that was never the case nor would it evolve into anything more than a scene from the movie, *'Step Brothers'*. If you have ever seen the movie, then this in some way is the perfect analogy.

All humour aside this is just another battle I still fight, another arm to PTSD that encumbers the mind and alienates me with thoughts of abnormality as a human being. It's these feelings and lack of self-worth or self confidence that drains your dignity as a person, I feel it is one of the reasons individuals with PTSD find it hard to come to terms with. It is so very easy to slip into a depressive state and it takes months, if not years of treatment, before you can digest and acknowledge the stranger things that haunt one's self.

Previously I spoke about my personal road to healing through EMDR *(Eye movement desensitization and reprocessing)*.

"The goal of EMDR is to reduce the long-lasting effects of distressing memories by engaging the brains natural adaptive information processing mechanisms, thereby relieving present symptoms. It is used to help with the symptoms (PTSD). When a traumatic or distressing experience occurs, it may overwhelm normal coping mechanisms. The memory and associated stimuli are inadequately processed and stored in an isolated memory network". *(Shapiro 2010)*

EMDR is not for everyone who has PTSD, but it has helped me to understand more of why I experience the sleep walking, flashbacks and nightmares. I guess it has in some way also help to put things into prospective and at least now I am able in part, to deal with the after effects in a positive way. Saying that, it doesn't take away the fact that these experiences are emotionally draining and can govern how a day, a week or even a month plays out.

The most important thing for me is positivity and to understand that I am safe and loved, that I have support and understand the importance of engaging in dialogue with professionals such as GP's, phycologists, psychiatrist's and family as and when the need arises.

I do recognise in the initial stages of PTSD or the precursor stages, for example: - depression, stress or burn out, it is difficult to express your initial feelings to anyone because you simply are not sure what is happening to you. There are no words and denial can be strong. Admitting you are on the fringes of mental illness can be embarrassing at first, a self-belief of personal inadequacy and the feeling of a world crumbling around you, are all common place and hard to come to terms with.

The mental torment becomes stagnant within the mind and has no way of escaping, so it was important to acknowledge I had a problem and to hold my hand up early.

'There is <u>no shame</u> in acknowledging the pain'.

Only the weak and blinkered are the ones that will ridicule and ostracise those people who feel the need to acknowledge a work related mental illness. Within the emergency service sector worldwide, some of those who now suffer because of the job they do, have become victims of poor or non-existent wellbeing programs and a management culture that has failed in its duty of care to employees.

The stories are the same, the pain is the same and more lives will be lost until those who have the power, recognise and deliver change. My inbox is full of stories from broken men and women who have written to me exhausted with systems that are constantly failing.

Not being listened to and taken seriously, inadequate therapy programs, insurance company ignorance, bullying, lack of support for partners and their families are just a few issues and only the tip of the iceberg. Some are left to battle alone and are left in financial distress, as well as having to deal with the knock-on effect and strain it puts on their family. If that's not enough.... now deal with your illness!!

It's immoral that serving or post serving emergency service workers should have to fight for everything that are profoundly obvious needs. Unfortunately, services see it as "just business" and will continue to penny pinch and make things difficult, detrimental to the very people that have given their all to a job and a service the community so dearly depends upon.

I am also aware that some services have had wakeup calls and are now starting to inject funds into wellbeing and support programs, which is at least a positive step forward. Better late than never, but too late for some and initiatives have come at the cost of human life.

My therapy was hampered time and time again as agencies employed by the service and those departments working for the service put me under continual pressure, trying to pin me down for dates to commence a possible return to work program. This heightened my anxiety to a level that hampered the work I was doing with my psychologist. It became harder to focus on healing and the set back on progress in my therapy was immense.

One example of this I remember was a pre-arranged meeting I had with a lady from a rehabilitation team employed by the ambulance service. I had met her a couple of times previously, I felt I had built up a good enough rapport with her and I assumed I could trust her. The day we met I was certainly not in a good place. I had been having suicidal thoughts for a couple of days and I was irritable and angry. She had been making notes throughout our meeting and I had asked if I could divulge some personal feelings and thoughts to her "off the record".

She agreed that anything that was discussed at that point would be 'off the record' as I had requested. I had literally poured my heart out to her, explaining how my illness had affected me and that I was not able to accept or consider engaging in a back to work program as I was fighting hard to deal with the intense therapy sessions. I was also struggling with a vast array of symptoms, associated with PTSD including an attempt at suicide. I discussed the meeting with Sharon on arrival at home and to be quite honest, I think she felt I had done the right thing by being frank about my current feelings and mindset. We both agreed that by being upfront with this lady, she may understand a little more about my illness and quell the pressure to push me in to a back to work program. Therefore, allowing me to focus more on getting better.

I later found out that an email penned by her had been sent to the ambulance service and their insurers accusing me of not being compliant and awkward. It stated that I was unwilling to make any attempt to return to work. Some may find this surprising but to me I felt betrayed and this tactic was at that time common place.

Blatant bullying/passive aggressive tactics supported by the departments within the ambulance service that profess to aid an employee with an illness back to work. My words of advice…. trust no one!!!

But I know first-hand that back stabbing and bullying did exist and is a cultural problem within the company I was employed to serve. The problem is the people that do the bulling are clever.

It's done verbally and never recorded or they use agencies such as the one I was involved with, to tighten the vice.

Insurers also employed by the ambulance service are terribly cunning in their dealings, forcing staff to accept pay outs when there fails to be a way forward in resolving a return to work. Generally, if it is a mental health problem the prognosis in returning to work can be poor. I accept all cases are different but in my case the job had affected me so bad there was no way I could go back. But in my final meeting with my insurer I found myself confined to a room for 6 hours with a lawyer. In another room, several people from insurers to ambulance service personnel sat around a table ready to have their say. It was at this point in my career I felt dirty, violated, useless and used. I was reduced to a number on a case file.

The pressure against me was unbearable. Ironically and a surprise to me, the email penned by the lady from the rehabilitation team was used against me as an ace up their sleeve. Thus, I was told, "if I didn't accept their offer they could force me back to work". The bullying tactics on show that day left me heartbroken and upset. I'd been backed into a corner as are so many.

Even so and over the last three years, I have expressed my concerns through the media how bullying within the ambulance service is rife. The CEO of the ambulance service I worked for shrugged his shoulders and is in total denial that such activities go on. In a recent event I attended, I was surprised to hear during a presentation by a senior executive, that such media claims had hampered and delayed the ambulance services move forward for change, after the paramedic deaths and subsequent internal enquiries. To be honest I was angered at what I was hearing. In my case I was standing up for others and fighting for change and for someone to stand up and admit they had failed in the duty of care of so many.

It seems in fairness that things are finally starting to move forward, and change is developing; not before time! I'm quite sure I have been forgotten about and that the ambulance service has moved on to other vulnerable employees suffering the same plight. However, the sad fact without a shadow of a doubt for the many changes, although welcomed; have come too late.

Too late for the ones who were bullied - Too late for the ones who were not listened to - Too late for the ones who were ostracized. Too late for the ones who sadly took their own lives!

It is also fundamental that the federal government recognise the need for extensive support for emergency service workers who suffer work related mental illness, just as they are doing for serving and post serving war veterans.

One thing I can be sure of is the day of reckoning will eventually come! The battle will continue and for those fighting day to day it is more important now to keep the faith and stand up for everything you have worked for.

But thank god for the people who run charities out there, helping those people in need. They work relentlessly year in year out offering support, fighting for employees' rights and raising awareness on their own time with minimal funds, which I think is amazing. They are our true guardian angels.

As for me!! I now believe in myself and I have come a long way in the last three years. From the brink of death, wallowing in the darkest corners of life and fighting mental torture, to a person who acknowledges an illness that now leaves me frozen. But I am back in the race to live a life that is abundant, happy and full of love and appreciation for those who believed in me. It was time for me to move on, time for change and to put the past behind me. My next hurdle was to find myself once again

Finding joy is probably tantamount to finding yourself and being comfortable in your own skin -

Morgan Freeman

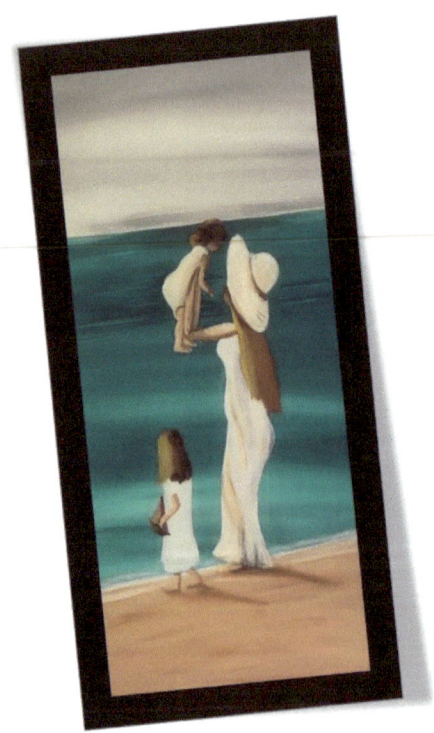

Chapter 2

West to East

After nearly ten years of living in Perth, Western Australia, the city that became my home since leaving the UK, had also become the place where so much sadness and heartache arose through my work. It was time to recognise my life and find out who I was again. It was the same for my wife Sharon, having been overshadowed and enveloped by my illness, she had battled alongside me for so long that she had lost direction as her own person.

Saying that, it seemed the right time for us to venture into new pastures. Surprisingly, there were so many of our friends who were also moving on to other towns or cities around Australia, it felt like a transitional time for many of us. All the friends we have, no matter where their hats would lay, always kept in touch They would always be there for support with a love that never faded. There was always that understanding between us all.

But you always leave loved ones behind, family, friends and colleagues. The same people who had been there for us throughout. The very people who had been a safety net and shoulder to cry on in times of need. We knew it was something we had to do as a couple to allow us to rebuild our lives. The ones we loved understood our need to move on and were extremely supportive.

Our children were always our biggest worry, although they were by now forging lives of their own. They seemed happy with their own worlds but even so, there was always a certain amount of guilt that bestowed the soul and a feeling of selfishness in leaving them behind. We had invited each one to join us in our new venture. For the most part, all were happy with our decision but there was a little resentment aired initially, which we both understood. No matter where we were, our door was always an open one and something that had never changed.

The love and support for each one of our children had never wavered in the slightest and as young adults, we knew that they were searching life's path for their own identity too. Maybe if they had understood more about what we had been through, it would have made more sense to them as to why we were moving. But there again Sharon had done a wonderful job in protecting them from the intimate details and only answering questions about my illness when questions were asked by them.

Sharon and I had spent many months talking about parts of Australia we would consider a move to, a place where we could breathe again. Each time it came down to Cairns, Queensland, simply because of the tranquillity and beauty it boasted. It would also be a place where I could expand my art and writing.

With Sharon's experience as a nurse, there was no issue with her finding work. I guess our main concern was the climate and how we would cope with the humidity and the possibility of cyclones, especially in the wet season.

We had visited Bali on several occasions, so we were aware how bad humidity could get and I had never experienced a cyclone, but to us we felt that was a small sacrifice to pay.

Preparation for our departure to Cairns was greeted with a dark cloud hanging over me, I was on a low due to a failed attempt to get back into the work place. I had attended a two-and-a-half-week cabin crew recruitment course and after arriving back in Perth, I began to realise that PTSD had won the battle again and I ended up throwing the towel in. Prior to that I had applied for many jobs but once PTSD was mentioned, companies did not want to know. Truthfully, I was still fighting with each day and the symptoms that hounded me.

My anxiety levels were at an all-time high once again and I was struggling to be around people. When all was said and done, on reflection, cabin crew probably wasn't the best career to apply for, still I felt as though I had something to prove. I was just nowhere near ready and am unsure at this stage whether I ever would be. It was still very much apparent that integrating with the public and socialising were still big hurdles for me as I felt smothered, anxious and irritable.

Furthermore, I had tested myself on a level that would have been unthinkable twelve months previously. A great achievement and a massive challenge mentally. It was something I felt I needed to do even though it was destined to be a bridge too far.

There are times when I prefer my own company, being alone in a more creative environment, painting or writing. I enjoy quiet times without noise or the hustle and bustle of life or engaging in activity that may cause triggers. To me, life is no longer an adrenaline fuelled race from A to B, but a time to heal, reflect and get to know who I am again and also who we were as a couple.

The big day finally arrived for the move and with our little dog Bella safely on her flight to Cairns via Sydney, I was soon on my way to embark on a new chapter in our lives. Sharon had already flown out to Cairns a week before to secure a place to live and to start a new job, so I was flying solo. My emotions were mixed, and I felt excited with tinges of apprehension.

I will never forget flying into Cairns over cascading, lush green hills, clear skies and deep blue waters. My first glimpse of Port Douglas below and especially the Great Barrier Reef was breath taking, shrouded with its coral islands glistening like jewels in nature's crown. Cruise ships and smaller boats, filled with enthused tourists were in abundance with visible white wash trailing behind each one. No photograph could do justice to the magnificent view I was witness to.

I could feel the weight of many weeks and months lift from my shoulders, as my mind wandered into a state of relaxation and contentment. My eyes welled a little as my plane landed and I just breathed a sigh of relief. Any worries I had now evaporated, any doubt I had was now history as I greeted Sharon outside the airport terminal.

Her embrace was warm and with a loving kiss I knew I was finally home. It was so good to see her as it had felt like we had been apart for ages.

Walking to the car I took a deep breath, absorbing the tropical ambience. The smell in the air was tangible, a mix of native plantation and fresh air. The hills were even more beautiful from the ground and looking up at them they appeared to embrace everything below. Guarding the town with prowess and providing a back drop so picturesque it was hard to believe. The humidity was apparent but certainly not over powering for the time of year, (July).

As Sharon drove me to our new home, I couldn't help but notice the vast fields awash with sugar Cain that stood tall and proud, blowing from side to side as the warm but subtle wind brushed their foliage. It was a far cry from the hustle and bustle of Perth! I couldn't wait to explore, and the thought of a new beginning filled us both with excitement. We were unsure as to whether Cairns would be home for us permanently, but at least for now we knew it was the right move for us at this point in our lives. We both needed to be able to breathe again, as so much had been thrown our way. Negative energy which had consumed us for so long because of my illness, felt immediately reduced and this move felt right.

With so much to see in Far North Queensland, it was hard to know where to start. We were living in a new area of Cairns close to Trinity beach, half way between the town and Palm Cove. Palm Cove is a favourite haven for tourists from around the world with fantastic restaurants, magnificent hotels and weekly markets directly on the beach front. Palm trees garnish the walk ways in and around the area which makes Palm Cove the tropical paradise people love and enjoy.

Sitting on the beach, small islands are visible in the distance and it's hard to believe when looking out to sea, that not far beyond the islands surrounded by its crisp clear waters, lay the Great Barrier Reef. This was something I had only ever seen on TV and in magazines and now this wonder of the world was in striking distance of our doorstep.

The beautiful town of Port Douglas was only 50km from Cairns, also with weekly markets full of people selling homemade wares, crafts, art and food. The quaint white church of St Mary by the sea perched on the water front a favourite and ideal place for weddings. Cafes and restaurants cater for every pallet and bulge with locals and tourists alike.

Cairns itself is a town that never sleeps! With night markets till 11pm every day, the fresh fruit and veg markets 4 days a week, hotels, restaurants, shops and a lagoon where families can enjoy an open-air picnic and swim till 9pm. Unlike Perth you can get something to eat up until midnight and there is a constant holiday vibe.

One thing that was apparent is the similarity in some areas of Cairns that are very influenced by Bali. Relaxed atmosphere, aromas and shops selling Bali styled clothing, families and friends eating carefree, sipping on beers and wines in the warm sultry evenings alfresco style. The dress code of each day, shorts, singlet and thongs. The only thing missing!! Bintang!!

There is pretty much everything in this part of the world to see and do from weekend trips to the Daintree rainforest, which requires a short cable driven ferry to cross crock infested waters. An eco-fest life style greets you on the other side which is totally deficient of Wi-Fi, internet and all communication with the outside world. The small pub that services the community is like walking into the pub in the movie 'Crocodile Dundee', with ice cold beer and relics of by-gone Australia littering the walls.

The tablelands, another area of Cairns, incorporates the small market village of Kuranda. This village sits high in the hills and is accessible by sky rail, cable car or by a long and winding road. Registration to a hippie life style is a must, or certified busker will suffice. It truly is an eclectic way of life up there.

Settling into the lifestyle of Cairns seemed to come naturally for Sharon and I. It wasn't long before we were into the swing of things and all the influences around pushed me to continue with my art and writing. I was determined to find myself and I felt it was important to discover who I really was.

Sharon was also starting to discover herself, away from the life in Perth we once knew. Now she was embracing a tranquil, slow paced life style which left time to think and reflect. In some ways, this can be a good thing, but on the other hand, having time to think, had allowed things to come to the surface within the mind.

Sure enough, lurking around the corner, was something that I wasn't ready for and would change the game completely.

She had been my rock for so long and now she needed me to be hers. Out of the blue, but hardly surprising another battle loomed.

"Each relationship nurtures a strength or weakness within you"-

Michael Murdock

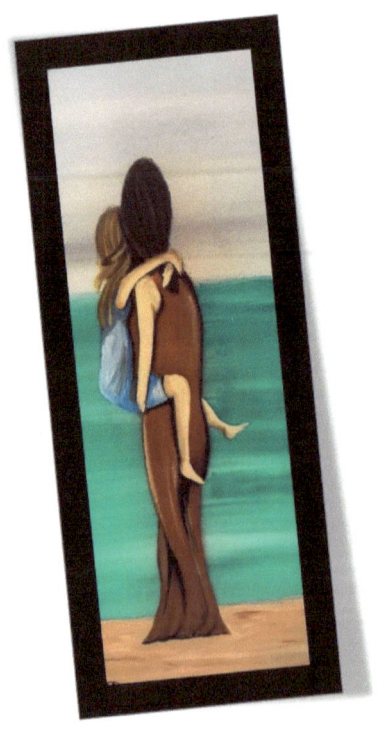

Chapter 3

My forgotten hero

Our new home backed onto beautiful, lush green rolling hills and we felt very lucky to be living in a beautiful part of the world. One day as we sat outside and reflected, a trickle of tears rolled down Sharon's cheek. That period of reflection between us and light conversation had triggered a sad moment, as she knew she had given her all. She was exhausted.

Her strength had always been something that had amazed me. She had always been there for me and remained loyal through the darkest of times.

The times my illness had driven us apart.

The times I had become unbearable and cruel.

The times I had deceived her.

The times I was unable to support or comfort her when she needed me the most.

The times I became angry, irritable and uncontrollable.

It was obvious that Sharon, my wife, my rock, my love, and my best friend was now trying to fight her own battle. The tears she shed were ones of anger, despair, frustration and the fall out of 3 years of relentless support and understanding.

Everything she had given; she had given alone with no support or help from the ambulance service. She was cast aside whilst I had battled and her calls for help were futile. I had always been her number one priority throughout my 3 years of my ongoing battle with PTSD. She too had been to hell and back. But these are the forgotten heroes. The partners of people suffering.

So, tell me who is there for them when she/he crumbles?

Who is there to offer guidance, support and reassurance for a partner?

When your own world falls apart due to PTSD or any mental illness, family support is so very important as I have said before. It takes a special type of person to fight the fight with you and for me I was extremely lucky. But the price the partner pays in most cases can be devastating for a relationship.

I have heard so many stories of relationships breaking down and indeed for an eight-month period ours did. We separated, and the sad thing is, the need for me to heal alone was endorsed by a certain professional within the ambulance service, even though the ultimate choice was mine. I was in no state to decide, but regrettably I realise now it was absolutely the wrong choice. It left her heartbroken. I would have given anything to turn back the clock.

All she ever wanted was her husband to be well. She wanted her husband back to the way he used to be. She wanted to be involved in my healing process. In her words "it just wasn't fair".

I look back to the day she realised there was something not quite right with me and as I explained in my first book, I had become an extremely angry person, irritable and worlds away from the person I used to be. I would snap at the smallest of things and arguments would erupt over situations that normally as a couple we could deal with.

If it had not have been for Sharon I probably would have carried on with my life, muddling through until eventually I cracked. I would have without a doubt succeeded in taking my own life. She always gave me something to fight for, something to live for, but ultimately, I was blind to the signs of a woman who just wanted to make things better. A woman who was crying out for help and support herself.

We also had a family and five wonderful children between us. Sharon had always allowed them to reach out to her when they became more concerned about my health. It was uncertain at that time just how much the children understood, but Sharon always put things in simple terms, something as a nurse and wonderful mother just came naturally to her.

During my illness, she suffered immensely and had watched me retreat into my shell. She was now retreating into her shell. She was witness to my darkest days, a verbal punch bag for my anger and I was witness to her tears, uncontrollable tears of desperation with her not knowing what to say or do. Constantly treading on eggshells, wondering whether to bring up a topic of conversation or to forget it for fear I would take it the wrong way and blow up.

My wife, a lady who has also dedicated her life to helping others in Emergency nursing, has remained dignified throughout. She supported me as a paramedic and the job I did. That support was unconditional. It is upsetting to note that the person who stands by anyone fighting a mental illness becomes just as broken and fights the same battle but in a separate way. Not only was she struggling to battle alone but her work suffered, having to take days off here and there and reducing her hours so she could care for me. In the end she ended up having to relinquish a management position due to the pressure I had put on our home life, it was too much to cope with and she was unable to focus.

When I look back now that makes me feel extremely sad but also showed how committed to me she was. But repeatedly I had no awareness as to what she had sacrificed to help me at that time. I was wrapped up in my own little world and my selfish ways, feeling sorry for myself and clueless to her wailing cries for help. It seemed no one was interested in providing her with the professional support, care and listening ear she so desperately needed. Not even her own husband could offer her comfort and reassurance.

Professional help and support may have been void in her need to understand; however, there were two fantastic people in her life that stood strong and were there to help and support her in the blink of an eye. These true friends, one Sharon calls her second husband and the other, solid and down to earth, gave their all. She had been friends with them for many years and had worked closely with them on a professional level.

It would be true to say that metaphorically speaking they were literally on call 24/7. She could depend on them no matter what and for that she was and is eternally grateful. She would have many heartfelt conversations with them and I have no doubt many views were aired. There would have been tears I'm sure but also an understanding that has kept them with an extremely strong bond to this day. One thing that Sharon mentioned, was that they had a code that would be brought up in conversation, something I thought was fantastic. Conversation would develop between them and then the question would be asked, "Is this a code Tangy"? Once acknowledged then it would mean there was need for a full-on face to face meeting and Sharon was struggling or had an issue she was finding hard to deal with.

Seriously these two friends are without doubt the most amazing people you could ever wish to have in your life. So many times their family lives were put on hold, to be by her side at the drop of a hat, no questions asked. It is extremely hard when life becomes tough, knowing who to trust and I am sure many of you have been let down or betrayed by people you thought were friends, but then shit on you big time when your back is turned. I can categorically say Sharon and I would trust these two-wonderful people with our lives. More importantly there would have been no way she could have gotten through without them. For all they have done and for all the love they shower us with year in year out, Thank you. Xx. For the record, Sharon still refers to you as her '*code tangy friends*'.

The move to Queensland allowed us to talk more and we could dissect the turmoil that we had left behind. Sharon still had many questions to ask me and it seemed now I was happy to answer them no matter how hard they were. Questions that would have caused arguments and walk–outs were now on the table and I felt comfortable answering. Anger and bitterness where no longer directed towards me but to my former employer. I know she would have lots to say to them but was it worth it?

All we wanted to do as a couple now was move on with our lives and distance ourselves from the months and years of hell bestowed upon us. It was time for new challenges, to meet new people and to pick up the pieces. It was time for us to heal and try to become the couple we once were. We were certainly in the right place to do that now. We were adamant nothing was going to stand in our way and we knew good things were to come. The strength of our friendship was becoming stronger and we were happy we had made it through to this point.

Over the coming weeks Sharon sourced help to talk about her feelings. It was in the hope that she could make more sense as to why she was feeling the way she did and to minimise the chance of things escalating mentally. One thing was certain and something she had expressed on many occasions, was the fact she had had enough of nursing. I think things regarding the job had become more strained and there certainly wasn't the passion and love for the job anymore she once had. Whether that was a result of what she had seen me go through or whether it was her wanting to protect herself mentally I was initially unsure. Things were becoming more apparent that the culture within the nursing sector, as to how nurses where treated by the public with regards to abuse and other forms of ill treatment, cemented her key reasons for considering a move away.

I was also aware that she similarly had to deal with her past nursing experiences. The bad jobs she'd been involved with had been brought to the surface of her mind and I think there certainly was a common ground between us. My illness had certainly made her analyse things more and I know she was starting to question her own state of mind. The pressure and the stress of dealing with me and her own issues were not going to be easy, but at least it was a start and now she could finally get the help she needed.

It still upsets me to think the pressure could subsequently have been alleviated had she been given or offered a paralleled support network at the same time I was receiving support. Again, that was never offered. I have always said that any loved one suffering a mental illness not only needs support from professionals, but the support from home is imperative to enable them to heal. This can only be done if a support network is offered to the ones who battle each day with loved one's suffering.

I am aware that charities are also now offering education and support surrounding mental illness. I think this is a wonderful tool for anyone wanting to learn more or use as a way of understanding. It is without doubt, something that employers within the emergency service sector should have been offering many years ago and I am sure now have, or hopefully are looking towards.

So, for us there is still more of the mountain to climb, but thankfully we can now do it together. A feat I am extremely grateful to be sharing with my forgotten hero.

The cost has already been immense but as with any team you regroup, re energise and push forward to hope and happiness. We could see the finish line but a few hurdles yet stood in our way and we were not about to be beaten.

Life for us had to go on and we had started to embrace new challenges together. It was a fantastic feeling for both of us, to be as one again. Having that time to reflect, whilst enjoying doing things together and exploring each other's minds, was like we were dating again for the first time. It was a time to rekindle, rejuvenate and rejoice.

PTSD had changed our vision on life. It had made us both value life more and we now had a 'just do it' mindset. Life was certainly too short and we were going to enjoy it to the max. There was still so much for us to see and do and we were grateful we could do it together. I still think about my attempts at suicide and what would have become of Sharon if I had been successful. It's one question I have never asked her and it's probably a subject I would never want to bring to the forefront in conversation. There is just no need I guess, but they are still thoughts I have. Knowing in my own mind it would have been devastating for her to have lost me and I dread to think how my family would have coped. That sounds quite an egotistical thing to say but does anyone think about it?

I can guarantee that no one really does, not until they have had a near death experience or have been on a downward spiral that could eventually have no other conclusion but to take one's life. Ironically, she had lost me during my illness and she was a broken loving wife for a long time. No words can express how hard things have been for her, the pain and suffering she endured may never be realised fully. Sharon is and always has been a very private person and I am sure some of her inner most thoughts and feelings will nestle in her mind forever.

Only the people that were close to us as a couple at that time could begin to comprehend and they know who they are. They too had suffered the pain of anger and feeling sorry for a lady and loyal friend who just wanted things back to the way they were.

I remember a conversation I had with one of her *'code tangy friends'* soon after I had come through the worst of the illness. The conversation was blunt, to the point and a real wake up call for me. She had pretty much asked me if I knew what Sharon had been through. Many other things were said during the conversation that hit home. That conversation made me think long and hard, but everything that was said that day was true and would never be spoken about again. The fact that she is someone I respect, made it a conversation I respect to this day and will always resinate deeply within me.

So as the tears dry, my hero stands beside me, head held high and shines with enthusiastic hope. Her positivity, love and affection continued to astound me day after day. Once again, she takes my hand, for which I am grateful and we walk life's path together. She once again is my safe place to fall and always will be my best friend.

There are so many people out there that will tell you, you can't. What you have got to do is turn around and say, "watch me".

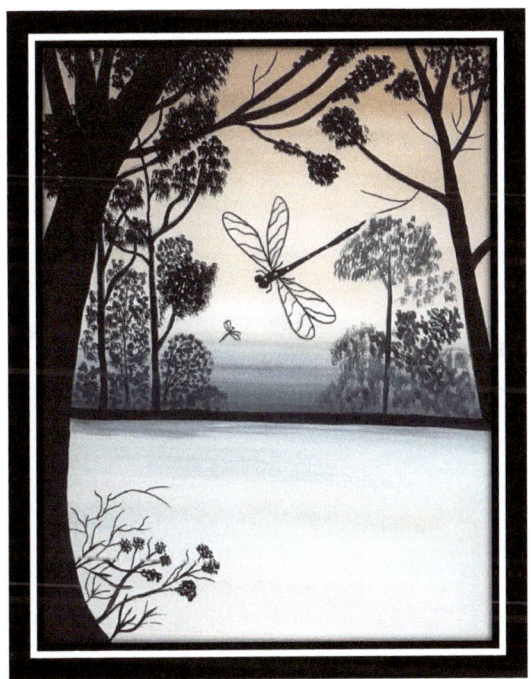

CHAPTER 4

DREAMS, THOUGHTS AND MOVING ON

Although my days seemed to be more manageable there were still times when I felt I was just not coping. My dreams were still haunting me and I found no solace at night time. I had worked extremely hard to eradicate the darker thoughts from my mind, even so there were still niggles I simply could not shake off no matter how hard I tried.

One dream that still repeats even to this day is the dream I have of being caged. The vision is very clear and I always remember that dream when I have woken. The dream takes me to a medieval time and my hands and legs are shackled. I am locked in a cage or prison. Straw lines the floor and there are people shouting but I am unable to see anyone. There is a distinct musty odour from the harsh sandstone walls around me. The ceiling is low so I am unable to stand. The dream itself never ends until I wake and when I do wake I sit up in bed shaking and scared, on the verge of tears. As I sit there in the early hours I feel very alone with an impending fear of doom encompassing my whole body. Sometimes I will climb out of bed to make myself a cup of tea to relax and make sense of my dream.

Other dreams are just as weird. For instance, one where I am standing in front of a mirror pulling out my teeth and watching them fall into my open hand. There were also days if I thought hard enough, I became very scared of going back to where I had started. Right to the very beginning of my illness, the point of diagnosis. As though for some unknown reason everything would just become undone again. Sometimes I would still have suicidal feelings, but not a feeling I want to harm myself, just a passing thought. I would think "would everyone be better off without me and has the battle all been worth it?"

So much carnage and upset has been caused by me, which leaves me feeling extremely sad. I guess the only person not going to take any blame for this is PTSD. He nonchalantly walks away to move on to the next. I would not wish this on anyone but unfortunately PTSD has now stooped to bestow its presence in less eager or unsuspecting hands. I was once asked in a therapy session "did I have a name for PTSD, given all the damage and hurt it had caused?" "The warrior's demise" I replied. We all strive in life to make a difference but those who give everything to help others, the true warriors of life can sometimes fall on the fields of courage having given their all.

Speaking of warriors, there was one little warrior in my life that seemed to make my days a lot more manageable, especially after a difficult day or night and that was our beautiful four-legged doggie Bella. She had been an absolute god send to both Sharon and myself. She had been there for Sharon during the period I was no longer around and had been a major source of comfort.

She could sense when things where wrong and certainly picked up on energy. Her trait was to jump up on the couch beside you and to push her head under your neck as if to say, "I know, here I am with cuddles, everything is going to be ok".

I have read a lot of material during my illness and so much has been written about dogs helping with people who suffer with PTSD. There now is an overwhelming demand for assistance dogs and I think the services who provide them do a wonderful job. She seemed to be a natural without formal training. We were just blessed to have such a wonderful fur ball that really seemed to understand. She always knew when I was feeling unwell and would follow me around the house. It was like she had a sixth sense. If I sat down, she would cuddle up next to me until she was happy I was in a better place. Generally, she would be spot on with her instincts and know when I was feeling better. It truly was quite amazing to experience this firsthand.

Maybe she understood my dreams and thoughts! Sometimes we would look each other in the eye, as if to get some reassurance for me, from her, that she knew. I often asked her to make it better and in some ways, she did. I always wondered what she thought of me and I know in the initial stages of my illness, when anger in me was rife and I flew off the handle about something trivial, she would bark and bark. I know it was her way of telling me calm down and maybe I should have listened to her more.

Her love for both of us was unconditional and she was a companion you could rely on. Stroking her made me feel much better and it certainly was a calming therapy in so many ways. Some days were so bad for me that she would just look up at me with those loving sorry eyes, which on occasions seemed to well with a tear. A watery acknowledgement that simply melted the heart. Her understanding continued relentlessly throughout the tough time Sharon and I shared. We were just pleased she could share our new venture.

My thoughts for the future were uncertain! Where we were now living in Cairns gave me the chance to think about, take stock of the path we had taken and reflect on the damage that had been done mentally to both of us. One thing was certain, I still needed help and now felt that I should continue with professional support with a psychologist. Sharon had also realised that she too would endeavour to seek help, she had to release the tension and demons buried deep within her mind and soul. Her approach to healing was always an alternative view and even though she was in the mindset that talking to someone would be beneficial, yoga, meditation and healthy eating were always top of her list when it came to heal within.

Our life style change and things were so much more laid back and on par with the way of life in Far North Queensland. Nothing seemed to be an effort, although nothing was ever done quickly here, that was the only downside. The culture here was very blinkered and it was hard to make new friends, so many people were here for short periods on similar transitional paths or just passing through. We were extremely lucky to have a group of friends already living close to us. We did spend quality time with them and they were a great support to us.

The one thing we did find was that the alternative healing culture was massive, so that was a big bonus. It was like a breath of fresh air compared to the hustle and bustle of a big city. There was certainly no hostility and you had time to think. I was happy to embrace our new life and was certainly up for the challenge of new things. There was so much to explore in this beautiful world of palm trees, sun kissed beaches, waterfalls and rainforests. It was like nothing we had experienced as a couple before.

In between our adventures, my therapy with a new Phycologist began. In our first meeting I noted she was a very sincere person, very welcoming and genuinely interested in the battle I had endured. She was originally from South Africa and had many years' experience in the psychology field. Slight of build, she sat in her chair with pen and paper in hand, listening intently to what I had to say as she scribbled away. There was agreement in the fact I needed ongoing support and I was asked what were my main concerns having come this far. I was blunt and honest and told her I feared a relapse. I was asked what did I mean when saying that? I told her about my dreams and that I sometimes still had suicidal thoughts but not that I wanted to hurt myself in any way. That I was frightened of going back to the beginning of my illness. Having come so far and achieving so much I still had a powerful sense that it would all just crumble around me. Everything I had worked towards in getting better would just evaporate, that was my biggest fear.

I told her about the heart wrenching, sinking feeling and sickness I would feel in my stomach when I thought about this fear. Then panic sets in and my body shakes uncontrollably trying to make sense of it all. Suddenly I realise it's not real, it's just a fear, the fear of losing, the fear of failure. I breathe and focus, and the feelings subsides, then I know in my mind it's all ok. Failure is not an option. Even so these were thoughts I would have on a regular basis these days, something I battled with.

I was told that these feelings were quite normal and that eventually the ideology of losing everything or relapse was nestled in the mind to help in the realisation of moving forward. Like a book mark in the brain so to speak. It was a memorial, an 'aide-mémoire' in the subconscious saying, "this is where you were! Now this is how far you have come and where you are now".

It made sense to me and the most important thing was to continue pushing forward and focus on the now and the future. After my meeting, this became clearer to me and I realised that my sessions were going to be based on a theory of keeping on track with my healing. The intense therapy days had long gone, and I knew these sessions were just really a safety net for me, a way of gauging where I was in mindset and mental wellbeing. I wasn't going to allow negative thoughts to dictate my future. In fact, I was so very happy I had come this far and I guess quietly proud of my progress.

My thoughts were also with Sharon and I was aware that she would also need my support. I knew I had to be strong for her whilst she dealt with her demons and set out on her own personal journey with counselling, getting the help, she so dearly needed. The help that was so long overdue. It certainly would be a test of my mental strength and I felt I at least owed her that after all she had been through. She still had a lot to get off her chest and I know she was hurting immensely.

Over the coming weeks and months, we once again worked as the team we used to be. We talked about so much and rather than life being one sided for the first-time, discussion and life experiences were a two-way street. The counselling sessions we embarked on were helping us to be open more together and that was fantastic therapy. This is how it should have been from the beginning. It gave us a better understanding about each other's feelings and we were able to discuss and debrief after our sessions. Thankfully, it wasn't just about me anymore. It was about us as a couple and although PTSD had been forefront in our lives for so long, it was time to learn to deal with it as a 'thing' rather than the big issue it had been. It had consumed so much of our time, so much of our life and we could dwell on that and let it destroy us or release from its grasp and move on.

The therapy Sharon was receiving I think was allowing her to open and release the anger and resentment within, but I know the scars of the past would probably remain for many years to come. I know I will carry a wealth of guilt knowing I have scarred the one I love for a long time to come. I had rubbed salt in her wounds for so long and now it was time for me to listen and be there for her.

There would not be a day that went by when I wouldn't think about this, to the extent it would profoundly frustrate me and sometimes end in tears. It was something else I would have to try and overcome, but I doubt it will ever be eradicated from my mind completely.

Many other things had crossed my mind over the last few years including the colleagues I used to work with. I still think about the job and I wonder how they are going. They will always remain in my thoughts and were a big part of my life. I have been asked on several occasions "what do I most miss?" I never have had to think twice and the answer will always be the comradery and the close family I worked with for many years. There were many characters amongst them and that's what made the job to be truthful. There were many times when moral was low and we all did it tough. Then like with any family we were there for each other and we just got it. We understood, we cared, we listened.

It's a strange feeling not to be part of that anymore and it is a sad thought. I still care for the ones who cared and I am still in distant contact with many. I guess sometimes I do worry about them and fearful that anyone of them could fall the way I did, I am aware that many of them have had to fight their own battles. Some have moved on to different careers, some are no longer with us and some remain, even so I am proud and honoured to have been part of their lives.

So, dreams and thoughts will always be part of my life, that's a given. Hopefully they will become happier and less vivid. My aim now is to hope and pray that like a bad headache, I will eventually get some relief from the intensity and diversity of them, that I can dream and think like a normal human being once again.

When we needed a hand, we found your paw and our little one that licked away the tears.

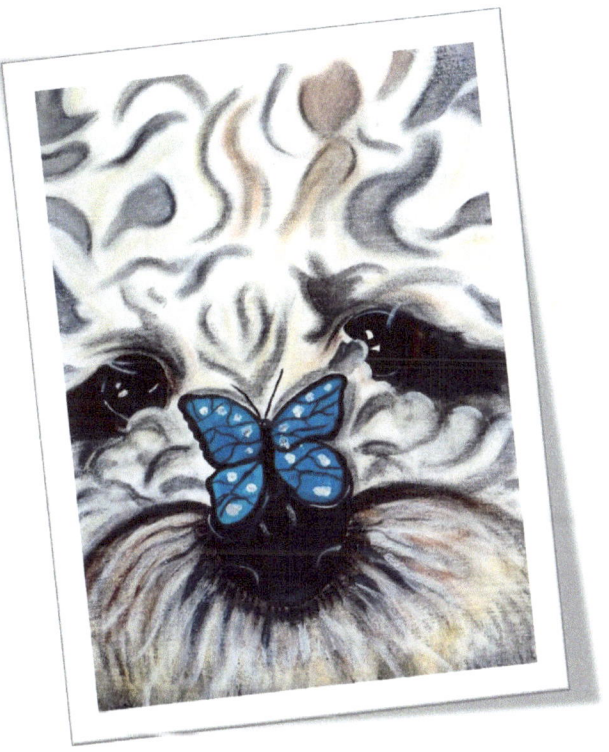

CHAPTER 5

SLEEP TIGHT ANGEL

We woke to a beautiful Mother's Day weekend. I climbed out of bed and as usual walked through the lounge area to open the back door, letting in the fresh air from the surrounding hills. I stood for a moment and took a deep breath, filling my lungs with the airs' ambient tropical fragrance. I had had probably one of the best night's sleep in a long time. I felt refreshed and happy to be alive.

It wasn't long before I was to be greeted by Bella our 6-year-old fur baby, who had just woken from her slumber and began tapping at my feet for morning cuddles and breakfast. As I looked down to acknowledge her, she briefly jumped up against my legs as if to encourage me to bow down and give her the usual tickle of her neck. "Good morning Bella" I said, naturally submitting to her demand. She was such a sprightly little thing and certainly knew her place in the household. As I had previously mentioned, she had been an absolute god send to us and we were so very thankful of her presence and of being blessed with such a wonderful little thing.

Her excitement rose and she skipped around the kitchen until finally I responded to her request for breakfast. Her ears pricked up as the biscuits fell one by one in to her bowl, followed by a licking of her lips. She was aware her treat was imminent. I laid the bowl in its usual place on the floor in front of her and she would perform her daily eating ritual. First, she would sniff her food taking only a small mouthful. Then she would walk away and approach the bowl from another angle. This would continue for a few brief minutes until she was entirely happy with what she had been offered. This was a ritual we were used to and there really was no rhyme or reason for her behaviour, it was just something we accepted. We had planned a relaxing day and after eating breakfast, discussed the possibility of venturing out to the hills. I think it was fair to say we were both feeling refreshed and relaxed. There felt no rush to do anything and we were happy just to take the day as it came.

As a family we had now settled into our new way of life and were feeling more comfortable. Sharon had undertaken a brief nursing post back in ED at the local hospital, but quickly realised it was not something she wanted to continue. The way things were done in Cairns were far removed from what she was used to. With some of the nursing ways in the department so questionable, it was enough to make her eyes water. Furthermore, she was never really welcomed as part of the team. It seemed the more prehistoric members were void of any change, and frowned upon unfamiliar faces. I think Sharon's eventual decision to put emergency nursing on the back burner for a while, was made easier and probably at that time the right thing to do. She needed a break from the dynamic environment she was so used to and to be honest, I would support anything she wanted to do.

Ironically and after much thought, she accepted a post at the private hospital working in mental health. I think she felt through experience with my problems, she was more in tune with mental health issues and quickly found it to be a less stressful and a more rewarding job. It was wonderful to see her come home from work full of vigour and looking less stressed about her work. She had met some wonderful work colleagues and before long felt she belonged.

By now I had started to explore my passion for art and writing in a more meaningful way. I was testing my ability in a way I had never thought I could. Although art and writing had helped me partly through my illness, was it possible to make a living out of it? Would it be accepted in the public domain? Writing Broken had certainly been a test on a different kind of level and it was more about therapy than sales, the sales were a bonus. The art I produced at that time was more of a communication tool and a way of expressing my fears and thoughts.

It was quite an exciting concept and one that was certainly supported by Sharon. She saw I had the ability and always said if you are serious and passionate then just do it. After all there was plenty of inspiration around me and it was time to challenge my creative mind.

Most mornings we would sit outside where possible and talk about new challenges and ideas for our future and today, Mother's Day, was no exception. With a full tummy of food Bella laid beneath us under the garden table, content in the knowledge we were by her side and her morning wishes had once again been fulfilled.

Heading towards mid-morning we decided to sort ourselves out and head out into the hills as planned. I remember showering and dressing as normal and once again walking back into the living room. My mind was focused on making sure Bella had enough water in her bowl, so I headed into the kitchen. I was mindful she was still in the garden so after filling up her bowl and placing it on the floor, I called her to let her know.

There was a strange feeling that things by her standards were taking a little longer than normal. She was a very inquisitive little thing and any rattle of a water or food bowl would generally spawn activity from her. Finally, from the garden door she appeared, but for whatever reason she seemed to be struggling to clear the step to enter the house. It took her a good few seconds for her to make her entrance and in disbelief I was greeted with a shocking sight.

It seems that she was completely paralysed in the one leg and was partly dragging herself across the floor. My heart sank and I called Sharon. Our first thought was that she had been bitten by a tick, so naturally I gently rolled her on her back to look for anything that may resemble something like that. We were surprised to find nothing and it was also strange to note she wasn't in any pain when we touched the paralysed leg.

In panic I called the local vet and explained what had happened and he talked us through another check for ticks. I told him there was nothing to see, so an appointment was made for Bella to visit him later that day. Unstressed, Bella made her way to her basket and curled up for a nap. We thought that maybe it was something that would pass, but still quite perplexed and worried, we kept a watchful eye on her.

Our day had now been put on hold and our immediate focus was on supporting the little girl that had supported and been there for us without question. At least half an hour had passed and slowly Bella woke and she made a concerted effort to stand and leave her basket. She was by now struggling to move at all and it appeared she was anchored to her spot. Again, she tried using her front two legs to pull herself forward. I moved closer to her at the same time and noticed that now both legs had given way and she was totally incapacitated to the rear of her body. By now we were frantic and extremely upset.

Once again, I called the vet to update him and we were advised to bring her straight to his surgery. The thought of anything happening to Bella filled us with dread and on the way to the vets, we both shed a tear. Sharon drove as I held Bella in the front seat in my arms. We had both noticed a change in her physical condition in such a short space of time. On the right-hand side of her body there seemed to be a significant swelling. Both having medical knowledge we knew this wasn't a good sign and naturally we feared the worst.

Arriving at the vets we were called into a room and laid Bella on the table. The vet examined her and asked a few questions. Our poor little angel laid there motionless and helpless, I felt sick as Sharon and I both welled once again. It was the worst feeling to see her laying like this, looking up with her sad eyes and wondering what was going on.

Then came the sucker punch, the news we were certainly not ready for and the news that would completely knock the wind out of our sails. His diagnosis was pretty much terminal, he told us he felt she had a cancerous growth that had burst, causing pressure on her spine. This in turn had caused the sudden onset of paralysis. We were devastated and could not believe what we were hearing. I think we both looked at him in the hope he would perform a miracle. There was a brief silence and I guess we were waiting for the options, but it was futile. Nothing he said would change the inevitable outcome.

The choice was now ours. Whether to have her put to sleep there and then, or take her home with medication so she could have a final night with us. We chose to take her home and cherish our final hours with her. We felt we owed her that but nothing could hide the fact we were heartbroken. We both questioned ourselves as owners…. Was there something we had missed or ignored? Had we failed her in some way? We knew the answer was no to all as she was our everything. She meant so very much to us. She was our baby. Unfortunately, it was just one of those unexplained things.

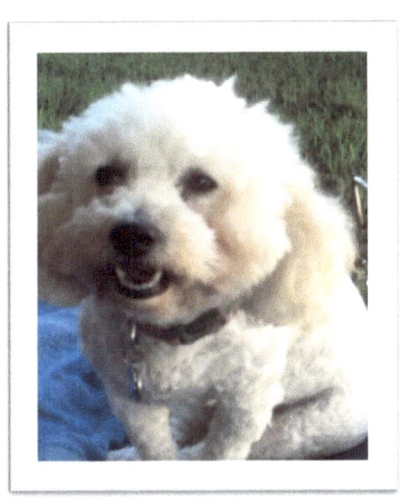

The last few hours before we say goodbye. She knew something was wrong and even in the end she still cuddled under my neck, to reassure me all would be ok.

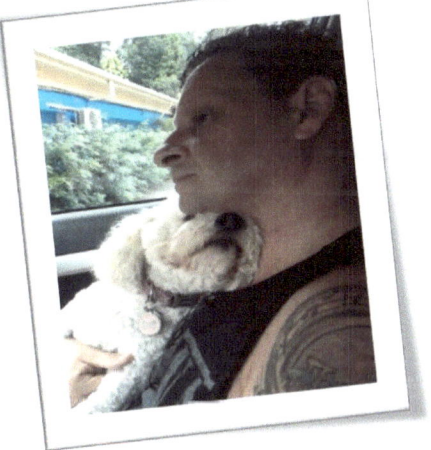

It was destined to be a long night and we made Bella as comfortable as we could. The sad and unbearable thing was the fact she could not toilet herself anymore. We had to predict the times she wanted to go to the toilet based on her whimpering but unfortunately, she was now in a great deal of pain, so it was even harder to gage.

Her basket was placed close to our bed, so we could be close to her, but it was impossible for her to lie down as the swelling on her stomach had now ballooned to an unspeakable level. We hardly slept a wink that night. Her whimpering became louder throughout the night and I recall getting out of bed on several occasions just to comfort her. It was truly upsetting to see her in such a state.

Dawn soon broke and we were both up early as we wanted to spend as much time with her as possible. I carried her through to the living area in her basket and to be frank, we were just going through the motions. There was no tapping at my feet for food with the same excitement she had had only the day before. We spent the last few hours cuddling her, crying and talking to her. I think if she was able to talk back, she would have told us she knew it was the end, and thank us for loving and caring for her. The sentiments were the same for us. Our little girl had been a pure rock of comfort and inspiration in the lowest ebb of both our lives. I'm sure anyone who has a pet can understand how loyal and caring any animal can be. They certainly become part of your family and the bond between human and animal is relentless.

We called the vet early afternoon to let him know that we were ready to bring Bella in, and I must admit that journey was probably, one of the saddest times of our lives. As we pulled up outside the surgery, Sharon held her tight and then passed her to me.

Just as she had always done when she was aware there was something wrong, she nestled under my neck as if to say, "It's ok daddy".

The ironic thing is she knew I was sad and upset but still she wanted to reassure me that all was going to be fine. We sat in the car and cherished our final few minutes with her. The tears flowed and we both felt for once in our lives, totally helpless to change the situation. I couldn't help but think had the strain and stress of what had happened in the last three years caused this! For a fleeting moment that thought certainly crossed my mind. I guess it's hard to know how pets deal with such things, but probably silly to think that it was a contributing factor. In times of grief and upset I feel things are mindfully over analysed as we search for an answer. The simple answer was that she was to be taken from us and her suffering would soon be no more.

The staff greeted us as we walked through the surgery door and they were fantastic with us. We were taken into a room and Bella was still carried by us nestled in her favourite basket. That's how we had decided she should part. We gave her one last cuddle as we made her comfortable in her bed. Her eyes watery and fixated on both of us. She looked so very sad and our tears for her were uncontrollable. It was heart wrenching to say goodbye as we stroked her soft fur and she was finally put to rest. Her eyes slowly closed as we both uttered our final loving words,

"Goodnight angel, sleep tight and thank you".

Our tears were once again relentless as we were left to touch and stroke her soft, fluffy body. She finally looked peaceful and was curled up just as she would have done, to sleep on any given night. Our little girl had been a truly, loving companion to us and although a devastating time we were so very grateful she had touch our hearts.

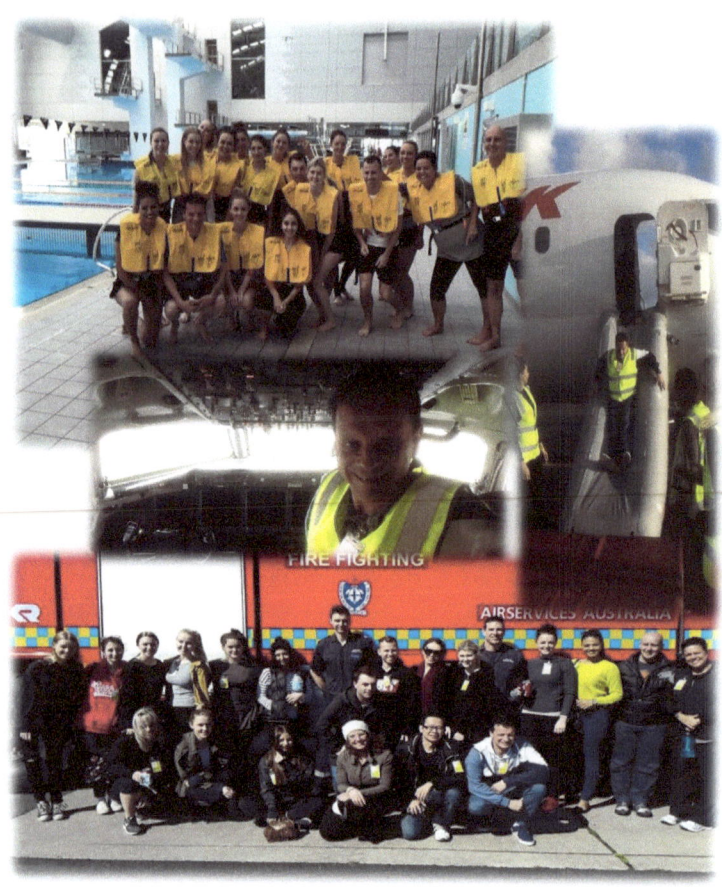

Cabin crew training with Quantas. My first attempt, since my illness to get back into the work place. Sadly, it wasn't to be, but proud of my achievement and blessed to have met some wonderful people.

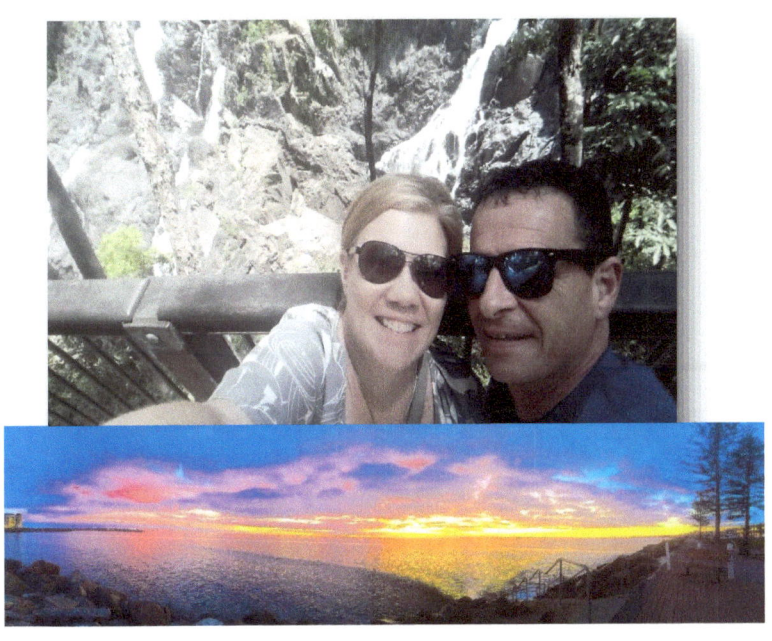

BEAUTIFUL CAIRNS, FAR NORTH QUEENSLAND

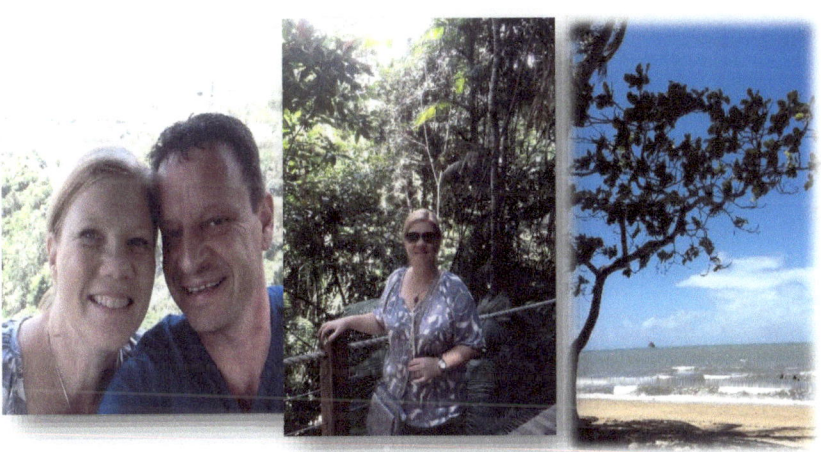

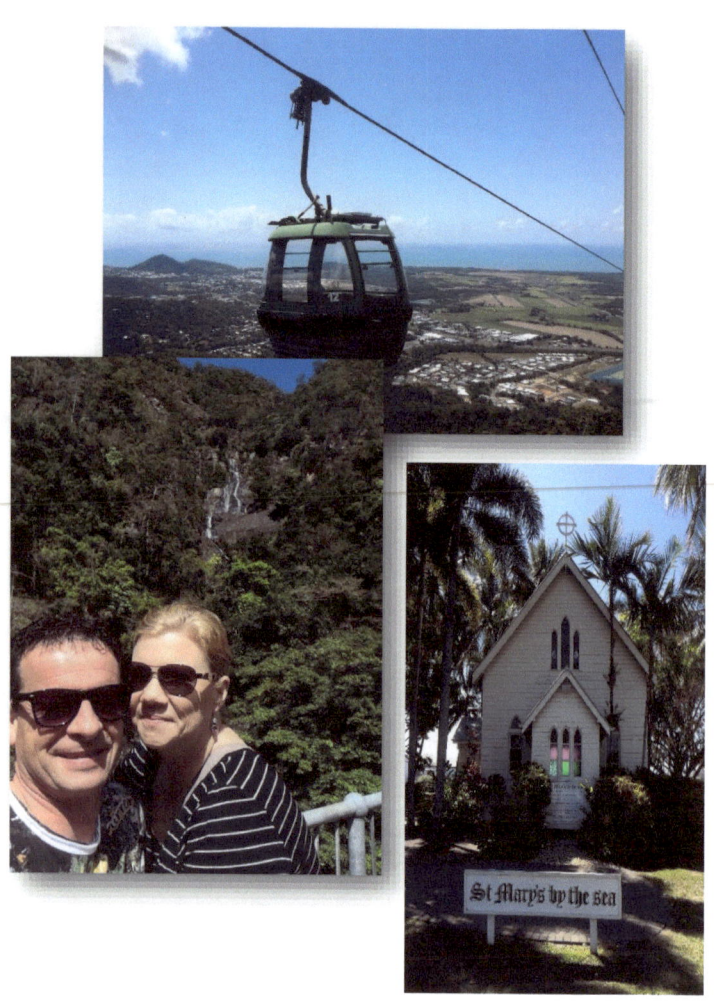

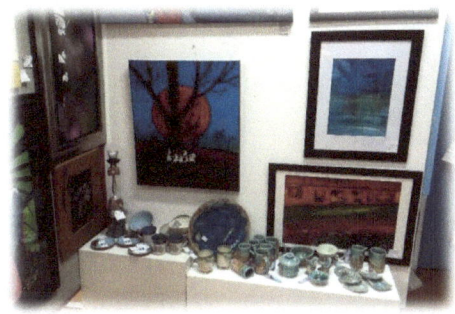

A proud moment – My art displayed

In one of Cairns Art galleries.

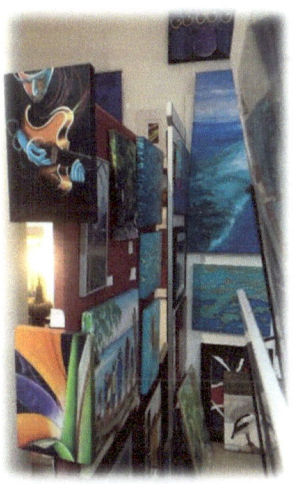

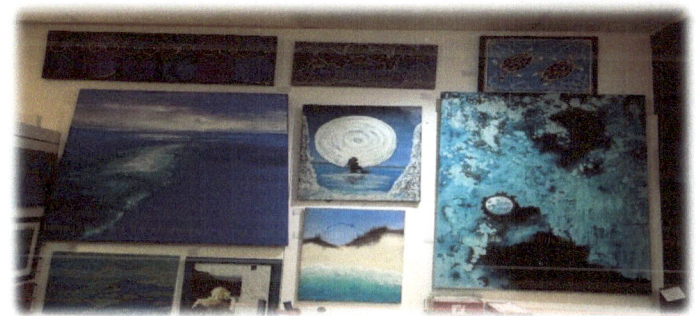

Ambition is to the mind what the cap is to the falcon; it blinds us first, and then compels us to tower, because of our blindness.

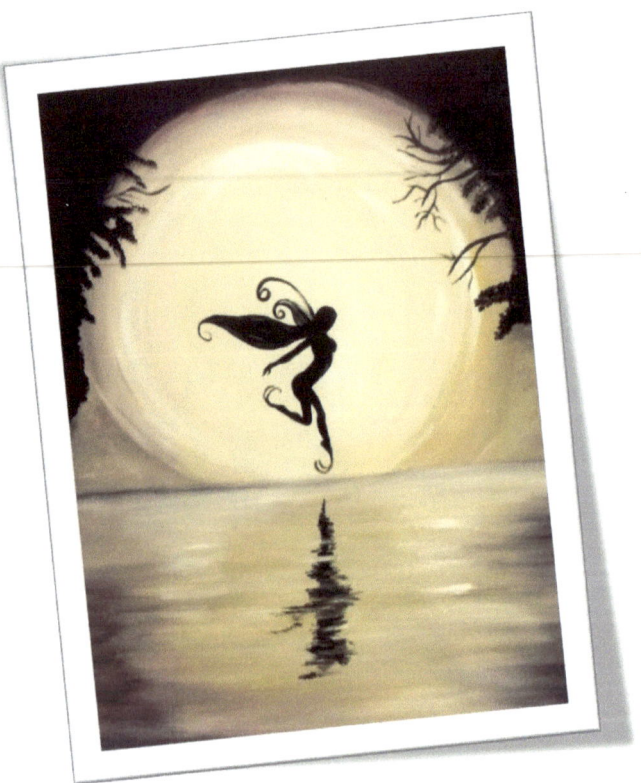

CHAPTER 6

A CUP OF AMBITION

The transitional period that we were currently experiencing was like a breath of fresh air. Our life seemed a lot less stressful and I was pushing forward with my art and writing, testing waters that would eventually decipher whether my passion and interests would allow me to forge a long-term career.

Sharon seemed settled in her work and with life in general, as things became more relaxed for her. We continued with our therapy and being able to talk about things with our phycologists. We continued with daily discussions between us, which we felt was the first time in a while we managed to start to understand each other more.

I now had several new art pieces that I had worked on and was looking for ways to push them into the public domain. By chance I was given the opportunity to have my works displayed in a local art gallery. For several weeks I had been looking at work that was out there which was so diverse and different to the art I was producing. I was now comfortable to show portfolios of work I had produced and was surprised when a gallery agreed to accept some of my pieces for show on a short-term basis. I was thrilled and it was the first time that someone who had been working in the art field for many years, saw the potential in things I had painted.

It was really the boost I needed and pushed me to continue producing more and more art. Furthermore, I had penned two children's books and incorporated my own illustrations. Things were starting to flow, finally. My book Broken was still spawning interest and I was invited by ABC radio to be interviewed about my experiences with PTSD. This came at a time when there was mass exposure in the press about how emergency service workers were being failed, wellbeing wise. To be honest talk was rife as more and more people had a story to tell about their own experiences.

Once the interview was complete I was approached by several more press agencies, to talk about my issues including ABC television. The ABC wanted to interview me about the subject of a bulling culture within the ambulance service. I was happy to oblige, as I personally had been subject to bullying and I was aware of how damaging it had been to others.

For many of you who watched the aired program it would have been apparent, it was an upsetting interview. At that time, I was extremely passionate and felt the need to protect my former colleagues. I admit there was probably an air of anger on my part and felt that my fallen colleagues had been failed. I, as with many others, felt that nothing was being done and things were just being swept under the carpet.

To be honest I think the program segment spoke for itself and that many of you would have had your own personal views. It certainly promoted discussion and highlighted the plight of those who had and are suffering.

I continued for many weeks and months working hard on my art and writing, which, in turn was helping me with my daily mental health battles. There were still many days I would lock myself away and either write or paint, sometimes speaking to no one other than Sharon. Socialising was still a big learning process for me and the days I did venture out were short and sweet.

Finding my niche in life was top priority along with learning to love who I was. Sharon and I were also starting to learn who we were as a couple too. We had missed each other and what we had. It truly was a wonderful and exciting time.

By now we were embracing life more and exploring our geographical surroundings, doing and seeing things we would never in our wildest dreams thought we would have. Although as I previously commented, Cairns is a strange place to fit into. There were lots of pros and cons about living there. Don't get me wrong it is the most beautiful and picturesque place we have ever lived, but its bloody hot!! Two seasons, wet and dry and when it rained it would rain for days on end. A fantastic place to find yourself and gather your thoughts for a period, but we knew it wasn't to be the place we wanted to live for the rest of our lives.

Over the coming months, we met some amazing people and made new friends, as well as rekindling friendships with friends who had moved to Cairns at a similar time. It would be true to say we were all at a similar pathway in life, soul searching and healing. We could talk as a group and were certainly there for each other in times of need. I think we all wondered what our next move would be. For our own personal reasons, we all wanted the same, but it was apparent that our souls would eventually part once again. We all had our own agendas and that was cool. That's what made us all special and we were happy that the universe would eventually answer.

As far as Sharon and I were concerned we needed to be somewhere we could expand our minds further and push our ambitions to the full. The move to Cairns had served its purpose and we were happy by now to consider our future for the long term.

During our period in Cairns some of our children came to visit and it gave them the chance to see a different part of Australia. Our trips to the great barrier reef probably one of the most breathtaking experiences and never had we seen the world through different eyes. The inspiration I gained personally was endless from a creative prospective.

For a few months my youngest son came to live with us as he too was struggling with his own challenges in life. It was destined to be a great tonic for him and was a chance to recharge his batteries and find himself once again. It's funny no matter how old your children are or how far away you are, they always come back to be with you, if only for short periods. It's always comforting and something Sharon and I always welcomed. Our door was always open and our love unconditional. In many ways we missed them being around and under the same roof, especially on special occasions. We missed the laughing and giggling behind closed doors, the hugs, the tears and everything else that makes a family a family.

There was always a sense of guilt at leaving our children behind, but our circumstances had pushed us to a decision we, above all, felt reasonably comfortable with. When all is said and done, if we hadn't of left Perth and looked after ourselves, then what good would we have been to any of them. We as parents had brought our children up to be fine, upstanding young people and we were so very proud of the people they became and are still becoming.

Over the coming months we realised that another move was inevitable, and we had come a long way in our mental healing. Soon plans were in place and a decision had been made for us to move to Melbourne. There had been lengthy discussions and we had analysed at great length where we saw our future as a couple. Melbourne quite frankly would give us everything we wanted. By now Sharon had realised that she wanted to continue her studies and her passion was in naturopathy. Queensland really wasn't somewhere that would have been able to cater for that and the way she wanted to study was to be hands on. Universities in Melbourne were in abundance and it was a passion Sharon had had for a long time. Completing her nurse practitioner studies was also an option, but her passion for nursing was waning fast.

The hospital she had applied to were happy to accommodate her practitioner studies and the bonus being it was a university teaching hospital. She was prepared to keep her options open and if anything would move with an open mind.

As for me, things were starting to open creatively and I was receiving commissions for my work and with Melbourne being the art capital of Australia, it was really a no brainer. I was now keen to expand and embrace my passion too. It really was the first time in a long time, I felt comfortable about what I was doing in life.

On a mental level with PTSD, things were better although the nightmares, unexplained dreams and sleep walking were things I was still battling with. I was just glad I had decided to continue with counselling and support because speaking to someone helped with the after effects. Although I was starting to move away from the reclusive existence and venturing out more, moving back to a busy city was going to be a big test, but a test I was ready for, a test I think we were both ready for.

With the move now completely finalised, Sharon soon left for Melbourne and with the bonus of her family being there, she had a base, living with her mum to start work. I was happy to stay back for a brief time and tie things up in Cairns, flying over to Melbourne for short weekends until the moving date. This felt good, it felt right, and we were finally happy to be once again starting a new chapter in our lives. With so many new chapters in our lives, we jokingly thought 'how big is this bloody book going to be!!'

But you know, when we all think about our lives, with the different stories to tell and all the experiences we all have in life, there are no guidelines. Some books are bigger than others, but I can guarantee that when we are both eighty, sat back in our recliners and pissing our pants, we can pick that book up and be satisfied in knowing it will be a damn enjoyable read.

"You will know you made the right decision; you will feel the stress leaving your body, your mind, your life".

Brigitte Nicole

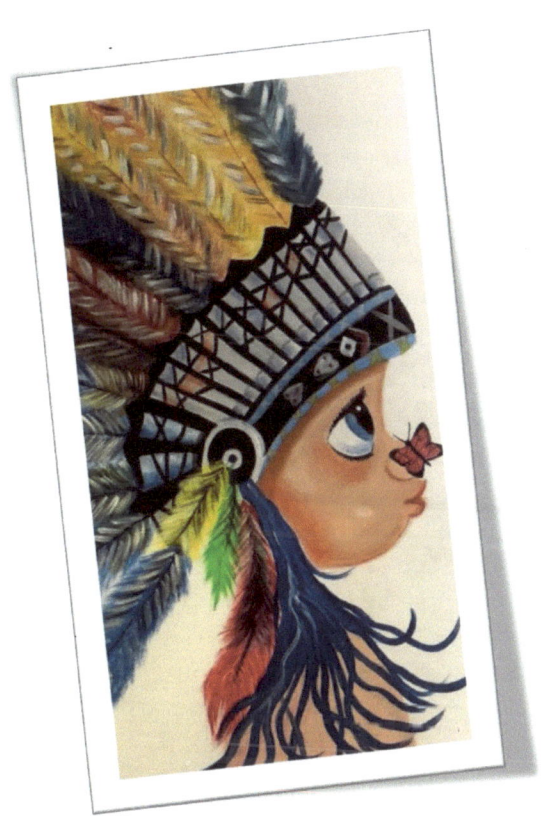

CHAPTER 7

SEVEN SEASONS IN ONE DAY

Our move to Melbourne was completed by early December 2016 and this vast city greeted us with open arms. It was bursting to the brim with activity and it oozed with culture. There was still an air of worry, wondering whether we had done the right thing, but I think we both knew that this opportunity would give us the stability we needed.

Melbourne was such a diverse city compared to anywhere we had lived and certainly a far cry from sleepy, hot Cairns. The skyline was so picturesque and seemed to change every time you looked at it. At night time it changed again and made it even more breathtaking. Its colossal Ferris wheel lit up with its flashing lights in the foreground, turning with delicate ease in the night sky and the city lights in the background, made it a magical site to behold!

We had decided to live south east of Melbourne in the beautiful suburb of Berwick, approximately 41km from the city. Berwick was very much an English style village, steeped in history and only a stone's throw from the local countryside. Its main street is lined with coffee shops, café's and restaurants. Trees that stand along the same strip were originally planted in testament to the fallen heroes of the first world war. Plaques were originally crafted to stand at the foot of each tree, but the plaques were never used.

Sharon and I moved into our new home just before Christmas and it was an exciting time for us both. We had also welcomed a new little man into our lives by the way of a four-legged friend we named Toby. He was a beagle-cavalier cross and was the most adorable thing you could ever wish to meet. Nothing could replace our Bella, but we did miss the company of a dog. Everything just seemed complete and we were a family once again.

It didn't take much time for us to settle and Sharon had by now eased her way into her new job at the local hospital's emergency department. Although nursing was not planned to be a long-term career anymore, she seemed happier working in a more professional environment. She had also decided to enrol in university to complete a degree in naturopathy as alternative medicine has always been one of her main passions.

As for me, well the healing process continued and I was now planning to continue with my vocational interest in art and writing. These were the two interests I now found were working for me and mentally did wonders. I was able to focus more on daily life and commissioned work was still coming in. I was at a point where I wanted to push the boat out further and see how my work would be received by the public. The thought of that was very much a scary thought, as still I had no confidence in what I was producing. Many people had said for a long time that I really should do something with my talent, but I wasn't sure I was ready. Maybe I would become a laughing stock, but if truth be known I wouldn't know until I tried.

I think because my early art had been used in my initial therapy to communicate, I found it as a private thing to me. In all honesty though, when I look at how it had helped me maybe it would help others. I love to paint for someone and present them with the finished article. The radiant smiles I have been witness to, truly warms my heart. Therefore, in some way, it still is a form of communication in that you are giving love, happiness and a part of you. How cool is that?

It wasn't long before a real opportunity came along for me to show and sell my art. I had found out just by chance that there was a very large local market close by that had been established for years. I bit the bullet and gave them a call to see if there were any vacancies. Whilst I was on the phone nervously waiting, I was thinking in the back of my mind, I hope they can't accommodate me! How stupid was it to think like that?

But you see in PTSD and mental illness that big wall is always available for you to erect. Or that excuse is always in the back pocket as a safe guard.... To get out quick. Suddenly there was a response on the other end of the phone, "Hello, yes, we have a spot for you this coming Sunday", the voice said.

Shit!! I thought, and it was only a fleeting thought, because within seconds my response was, "Ok thank you see you then". Oh my god, I had done it! This was the biggest leap of faith for me in 3 years. I'd committed to showing and selling my art. Then I panicked, what if I don't have enough work? What if people hate what I have painted? What if I lose my shit??

"Now focus Chris" was Sharon's response and she put things into prospective. At the end of the day I had nothing to lose and certainly nothing to lose by trying. Then I became excited at the thought. For the rest of the day my mind played tag, Its good, its bad, no its cool, so on and so forth. Then the sleepless nights, the over analysing, the doubts... until the morning of the first market came!! I think I drove Sharon crazy for the best part of the week.

I left home on market day around 6.30 am, having not slept much at all. I'd pretty much tossed and turned most of the night and was running on adrenaline. I was extremely anxious at not knowing what to expect. It was the first time I had ever done anything like this and my expectations were mixed. On arrival I was allocated a small stall, only 3 meters in length and fortunately I had a back wall which would enable me to hang some of my paintings. I was greeted by several other stall holders, all curious as to what I was selling. Their comments regarding my work were very encouraging. An older chap shook hands with me and welcomed me into the fold, which broke the ice and gave me some reassurance. I wouldn't say that I had any plan or structure to how my work was displayed but felt happy at least I had come this far.

Once I had set up my stall I decided to wander around to see first, if I had any competition art wise and second, to get a feel of what was on offer. The market area was vast with 4 indoor type hangers one of which I was in. On the outside there were people selling homemade crafts, fresh fruit and vegetables, jams, cheeses, clothing etc. You name it, it was all there but no one was selling art!! This was good and gave me a great boost, because if I did well here then I would be happy to stay on a permanent basis. It was all very exciting, and I felt strangely enough at home. This is where I wanted to be and something I had wanted to do for a long time. I was humbled by the response and comments I'd initially had from stall holders around me, so maybe I was on the right track after all.

Soon customers started to stream in and as they passed my stall they stopped, looked, pointing at various works and smiled. It made me feel relaxed and just the smiling from their faces alone was enough to reassure me that my work had hit a note in their minds. I'd made myself some business cards on the cheap and anyone who showed interest was offered one. It wasn't long before people approached me and started asking me about my art and some of my books I had on display. I had a few copies of Broken and next to that a little description about the book and why I had written it. It seems the book was receiving a lot of attention which surprised me. The ice breaker and my first sale came from a lady who first picked up the book, read my book's description, looked at me and said, "can I give you a hug"?

I looked at her a little perplexed but naturally bowed to her request. What harm could a hug do!! She walked around to the side of my stall and as I approached her, she hugged me tight and burst into tears. As we broke apart she simply said to me "thankyou". As she held my book in her hand, briefly shaking it she said to me, "you have no idea what this means to me, thank you so much for writing this and for telling your story". I was a little taken back and she proceeded to tell me that she was a paramedic, recently diagnosed with PTSD and had attempted to take her own life several months ago. She was now struggling with getting herself well and fighting with work cover and other agencies. She told me she felt that nothing was going well and her relationship with her family had broken down. She thanked me once again after purchasing my book and parted with a tentative smile.

I sat there for a moment and felt truly humbled, then thought to myself that since writing the book, I had never met anyone personally that had bought one who was suffering. To see face to face and first hand a person who felt my work could make a difference to their lives was mind blowing. Sure enough I have had lots of feedback through social media and via text and email, but this felt unbelievable.

My body was trembling and for a moment I forgot where I was. My eyes started to well and I was struggling for a split second to control my emotions. My throat became sore as I tried hard to push back the pending tears. You know that feeling when you really don't want to cry, and your throat starts to hurt? I didn't know what to do, where to look. It was like looking in to a mirror of myself 3 years ago when the lady stood in front of me. I felt so very sorry for her and I totally understood what she had still to go through. The sad thing was I could do nothing to help her. A few reassuring words of kindness without being patronising was all I had.

The morning moved along as I dried my eyes and focused on coffee and people watching. It's hard to judge what people like art wise as it's such a personal thing. My main gauge was to look at T- shirts people wore and things they were purchasing from other stalls. This always gives a wonderful insight as to what interests' people and makes them tick. My work was extremely eclectic, and I had tried to cater for all tastes however, my books seemed to be attracting more attention.

By midday I had sold 4 books, a small painting and had a commission, so I was extremely happy. Lots of people came over and talked to me about my work and there were some wonderful comments. The morning had flown by a lot quicker than I expected. Some of the other stall holders had enquired as to how my day had gone and had I enjoyed it? I just felt so at home here and all the worry had passed. There really wasn't anything to worry about in the first place and there was no doubt I would be back.

When I arrived back home I felt relieved, content and emotional but most of all, thrilled I had taken that first step. Sharon was so happy for me and extremely proud. I think it was something I had to prove to myself and I guess a bookmark in my mental state that for the first time, Sharon could physically see. She could see progress in my healing and another barrier had been demolished. I was so very thankful for her support once again and maybe, just maybe I could do this. I was pleased my work had been accepted publicly and it was now time to grasp that opportunity with open arms and embrace the hell out of it.

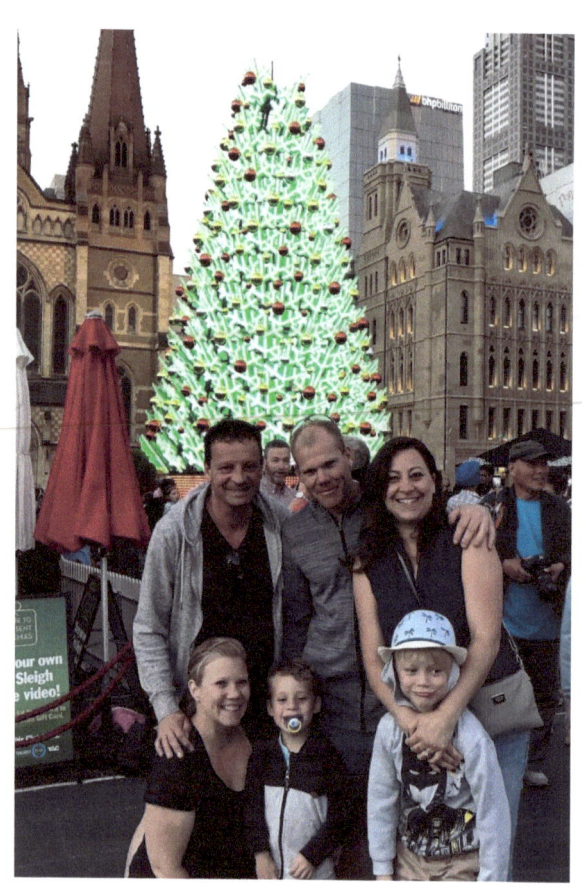

Our Melbourne family.

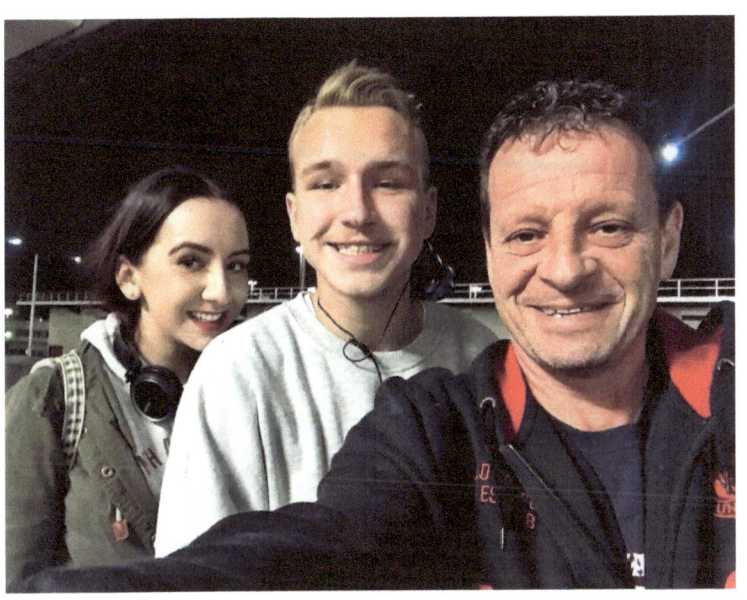

With my children on a recent visit to Melbourne.

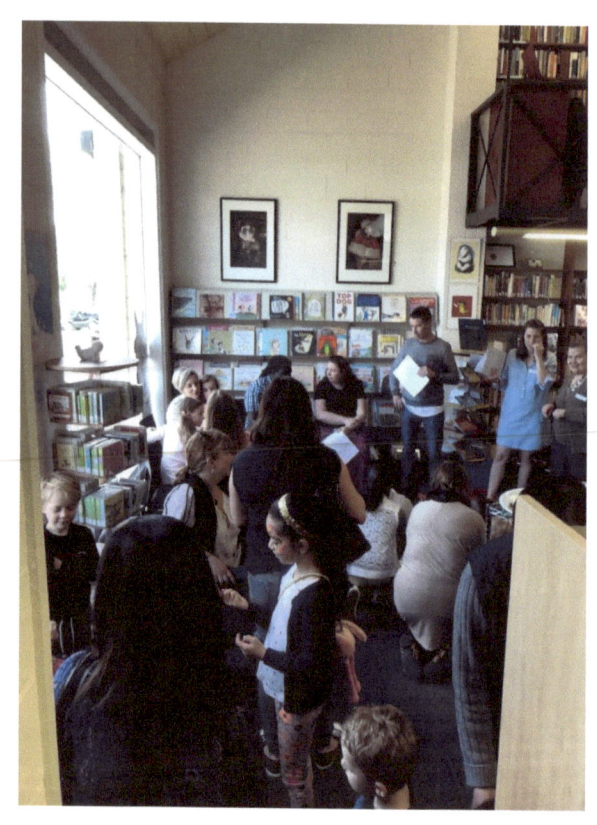

Children's book release morning for 'ROCKY THE ROO' in Berwick, Vic.

Art is not always about pretty things. It's about who we are, what happened to us, and how our lives are affected.

Elizabeth Broun

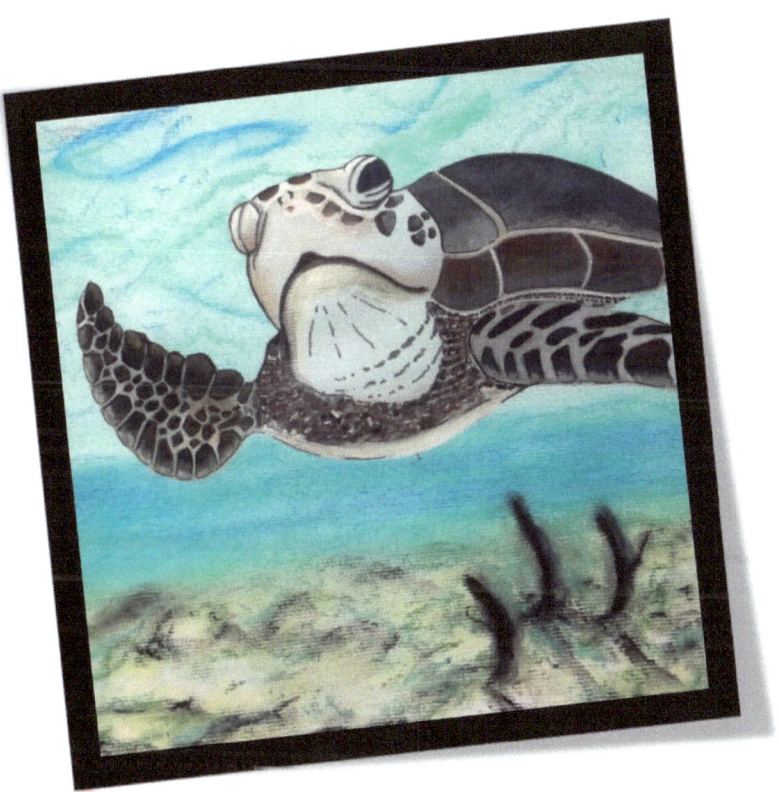

CHAPTER 8

ART THERAPY

Art is the meeting ground of the world inside and the world outside

As the weeks passed things were starting to come together. Settling in Melbourne had become easy for us both. I was touching base with a new GP who was very understanding and supportive of what I had been through. She was so very easy to talk to and encouraged me to continue with my vocational work and focus on using the tools I had to get me through each day.

Sharon had now started her studies in Naturopathy and was making weekly visits to university in the city by train. She was totally focused on what she wanted out of life and to be able to follow her passion, was totally what she needed. She also needed Starbucks too, which apparently is just outside the station on her arrival in the city. She calls it her happy place and who am I to argue with that!!

Spending time with extended family who live here was a wonderful thing and it was also great to see the children who liked to come and visit. It allowed them all to see yet another part of Australia and I must say that I think Melbourne was top of their list so far. There is never a day or week where nothing happens and most times we are so spoilt for choice. We have spent lots of time perusing and exploring this fine city, trying new cuisines, shopping and generally enjoying everything it has to offer.

The comparison to my home town of Manchester is uncanny with its old tram system. Maybe that's why I feel more settled here!! Not just because of the trams, the people seem more accepting and customer service certainly makes shopping a lot easier. I don't feel as stressed, although I still must be cautious as to knowing when enough is enough.

One scary incident came during our first Christmas at one of the big shopping centres near our home. It was boxing day morning and my daughter was staying with us. It was decided to go to the sales as we had not long been in the house and on the lookout for bargain furnishings. I was a little sceptical but thought, "ok let's do it!!"

The shopping centre is on several floors and serviced by escalators up and down. The store we wanted to look in was on the ground floor and I was surprised that it really wasn't too busy. Mind you it was only early in the day so hopefully we would be in and out before the hordes of people descended. We managed to get what we wanted relatively quickly but with sales on there is always something else you see and want to look at. After about an hour I was beginning to peak and Sharon had recognised I was beginning to fade. It was starting to get busier so she told me to head back to the car with my daughter. This was the first time my daughter had seen me like this and naturally after a little explanation from Sharon, she was happy to assist.

We headed to the escalators we had come down to find them out of action. Seeking another way out we moved to the next set a few minutes' walk away. To my shock they were also out of action. By now I was sweating, and the mall was filling with shoppers quickly. We frantically searched for lifts with my daughter keeping her cool and guiding me. We couldn't find them and by this time I was shaking and felt quite sick. I felt trapped as people came from all directions. The sweating became worse and my hypervigilance was now at an all-time high. I just wanted to get out as I was finding it hard to breath. I pulled all the tools out of my mind to help me through. Looking down at myself, I wasn't injured, I wasn't bleeding. No that's not working…. and the kid screaming behind me from Christmas overload was driving me mad. In fact, there were several kids suffering the same…OMG!! Nothing seemed to be kicking in, what the fuck?!!

Then you think the worst and start looking around for a reason for feeling trapped. Why are the escalators broken? I'm now in shut down mode, my daughter by this time had taken control and calls Sharon. I'm frozen to the spot. Within minutes I see Sharon and was reassured, then guided to the nearest lift. The same lift we had passed several times earlier. I can't tell you how happy I was to see the car and can categorically say, boxing day shopping is well and truly not a clever idea if you have PTSD.

This Christmas was a standing joke between Sharon and I as we watched TV and the adverts for the sales came on. "You up for it"? she says, with a smile on her face. My reply...!! "Bollocks".

Week in week out I was now getting into the swing of the market thing and I was getting that busy my poor little stall was bursting at the seams. Orders were coming in thick and fast. My books were selling out and although I was pleased as punch, it made me excitedly nervous. People were liking my work and coming back for more and more. Before long I requested an extension to the stall I had and within a short space of time it was granted to me.

The people that were running the market obviously saw I was committed and I was bringing in new custom. It wasn't long before I was well and truly welcomed as part of the market community and word was getting out locally about my talent. Business owners from local café's and shops were ordering paintings. A lady from the local library offered to run a book signing for one of my new books, which took me by surprise. I had never imagined a book about a bush Kangaroo would attract so much attention, but the day of the launch saw mums and dads with children pushing to get in. The smile on Sharon's face that day said it all. She was so proud and she really enjoyed it. She looked at me as if to say, 'you made it here'. Another funny thing she still says which is total sarcasm.... "There's nothing here for you though is there?" This was in reference about a mini breakdown I had prior to our move and my dummy spit during a conversation about moving to Melbourne. I just said to her, "there was nothing in Melbourne for me". I think the initial thought of moving again at that time had just gotten the better of me and I felt over whelmed.

Later in the year I was approached to attend the annual paramedic symposium which was to be held in Melbourne. I was asked if I would do a presentation on art therapy in PTSD as a guest speaker and how it had helped me. I felt truly honoured but a little anxious. There was no real pressure on me to attend and the choice was mine. After much thought I decided it would be good for me and may probably help others. I had never stood and spoken in public before about my illness, but I felt if I can publicly now show and sell my art then why can't I do this? I accepted and a week before the event I was emailed the running list of other guest speakers. I swallowed deeply as I read the list which included CEO's, professors, doctors and several other research academics.

I knew in my own heart of hearts I had to do this. I wanted to get my story across and this was probably the best forum and chance I would have of doing that, art therapy and writing had played a big part in saving me. It was a subject I passionate about and felt it was something that may be of alternative help to others who are at breaking point.

When the day finally came I was introduced to an array of people who seemed happy to see me. There was a lot of hand shaking and nerves but with Sharon by my side I was feeling relaxed. I'm sure she was feeling a little nervous for me but she took it all in her stride. There was one other person that did turn up to support me, I had been chatting to him for some time. He, himself was a seasoned paramedic, no longer in the job and had suffered immensely on a mental level. He had been a great support of my art and writing. When I told him what I was doing he said, "Chris, I'll be there cobber, wouldn't miss it for the world".

Sure enough within minutes of my arrival, he walked in. A man of his word and a true-blue Aussie. It was the first time I had met him face to face and it was like we were best of mates, cracking jokes and most of all making me feel at ease. I was so grateful to see him and that was a touch of gold that meant so much to me.

The day kicked off with introductions and lots of talks on wellbeing and statistics. It was an excellent insight as to how wellbeing in mental health was developing and was nice to see people who were working so hard in the wings, to make the work place a safer environment, talk with enthusiasm. The morning unfolded, I felt, quite quickly and I was due to do my thing after lunch. As the time got closer, I began to shiver a little in anticipation, but I was ready. I was at the point of no return and I felt prepared.

I had prepared myself a speech, to ad lib was not one of my forte's and I had never once spoken publicly in person before. The lunchtime break was a bit of a haze and I didn't really feel that hungry. Once again, I mingled and was introduced to people who anticipated my talk and were pleased to meet me. Again, I felt at ease although I knew this was going to be a real test of my mental stamina. I think the biggest thing I was worried about was breaking down, crying in front of everyone or even just drying up.

I'm sure if that happened people would see it for what it was, and I know many there were aware as to what a massive thing this was for me personally. As I sat in my chair with speech in sweaty hands, my introduction was announced. I looked at Sharon and smiled nervously, walked down through the auditorium to take my place at the podium in front of the audience. I looked up and thought, "shit!! This is it!", as I shook slightly on the spot. All eyes were now on me. I paused, looked up once again and introduced myself. The room fell so quiet you could hear a pin drop. I swallowed deeply, took a deep breath and I was away.

Everyone listened intently to what I had to say as my art work was projected on the wall behind me. The silence was palpable and I wasn't sure if that was a good or dreadful thing. I kept going, remembering to fill my time with deep breaths and pauses, allowing the audience to absorb my words. So far so good. Then there came a point I could feel my throat quiver, the pain in my throat. I knew what was coming next and thought shit, no, as I tried with all my might to overcome the emotion. The next sentence I spoke was the hardest and I had to stop, mid-sentence, to take a deep breath and compose myself. 'Please, please not now' I thought to myself, 'don't cry!'. I breathed again, I looked up and thankfully, the pain in my throat stopped and I was able to continue.

Nearing the end of my speech, I was feeling easy and relieved as the final words echoed to the back of the room. I looked up and the room burst into rapturous applause, 'I'd done it!' It seemed my speech had been an overall success and was greeted soon after by lots of people congratulating me on a heartfelt and powerful talk. I felt great and at the same time quite humbled, but my hope was that maybe, just maybe, someone would take away my words and those words, may help them turn a corner in their own personal struggle.

For those of you who were not able to attend or see my story in paramedic Response magazine, Spring edition, here is the speech in its entirety.

I would personally like to thank all those involved, who gave me the chance to stand up and talk that day, it meant so much.

Art therapy in PTSD: How art therapy has helped me in my battle with PTSD- my Plan B.

Overview:

PTSD for me led to withdrawal and disconnection from society, friends and family. It was imperative the root cause of my illness was identified to provide the appropriate therapy, care and support needed to aid in my recovery. But one to one discussion alone during therapy led to verbal suppression. Speaking about traumatic events would invoke upset, embarrassment and a slide into a depressive state. I found it at times extremely hard to express how I was feeling. It was therefore important for me to sometimes non- verbalise traumatic work-related experiences by way of supplementing my wellbeing and healing process with art therapy as a way of limiting the loss of connection between myself and others. Art therapy helped me exercise my mind and soul, which in turn made expression about traumatic events easier. The benefits of art therapy in my case and the use of creative skills were profound and being allowed to embrace this therapy as part of my healing process was crucial to my care.

Good afternoon everybody and it is an absolute pleasurer for me to be invited as a speaker here today. For me this is a big ask to stand here before you and is also my first ever public presentation which allows me finally to be open about my art and how it has helped me through my personal battle with PTSD.

My name is Chris Mawson, I am a former Paramedic of St John Ambulance, Western Australia and Author of the book, Broken, a paramedic's battle with PTSD.

My story starts back in October of 2013. I had actively been working as a paramedic in Perth, Western Australia since 2007 and previously in Manchester, UK. I was passionate about my work and fully committed to making a change to people's lives. In a nut shell, it was my dream job, full of excitement, pumped with adrenaline and diversity. I was being paid to save lives. But as with any dream, the bubble burst and I personally hit the ground with a bang.

In October 2013, my life changed for ever after near 18 solid months of horrific jobs- from hangings to road traffic deaths, murders and being personally assaulted with knives, not forgetting the tragedies I had seen during my 15-year career, it finally came to this- one traumatic and upsetting job during a nightshift. The one job that catapulted me into a world totally alien to me.

A world void of understanding or compassion and as I sat there, lying wounded next to me was the empty shattered shell of the person I once was…. The caring paramedic who had given his all to others was now fighting to care for himself. I had now locked horns with PTSD and it wasn't about to let me go without a battle.

PTSD was going to make me pay for all the good I had done for others?

But Why me? Why choose me?

I had been brought up by loving and caring parents who had passed down their caring ways to me. I had served my Queen and country as a bandsman and infantry soldier. I have 3 beautiful children and most of all a loving wife, Sharon, who I am pleased to say is here today and has stood by me as my rock. Life had been truly good to me but still I could not understand why PTSD had chosen me.

Once I understood what PTSD was I felt angry and let down. In my eyes, there was no duty of care and my wellbeing had now suffered. The signs were there but as a paramedic you think nothing of the potential damage this line of work can do to you. You continue week after week, servicing a community that needs your help.

I needed a plan B and I had a choice. These choices came after deep thought and intense soul searching over weeks. In no order, these were the choices I felt I had –

Alcohol

Drugs

Suicide

My state of mind at that time could focus no further than the 3 afore mentioned choices until my wife suggested I seek professional help. The night sweats, flashbacks, hypervigilance, anxiety and anger towards those close and dear to me had started in earnest. She was more aware of that, being an ED nurse for many year, and it was at that point I approached the ambulance service. I sought the help I needed through therapy with a clinical psychologist who specialised in EMDR- EYE MOVEMENT DESENSITIZATION AND REPROSESSING.

Something I am sure a few people sitting here today will be familiar with.

It certainly does not work for everyone and is certainly a contentious subject in some circles, but for me, after 12 months of exposure to its powers and other elements of psychology support, 'The real plan B was much clearer'.

CREATIVITY was my plan and in my case, it was Art.

A common occurrence for me after experiencing so much trauma was a hesitancy or inability to discuss the incident out loud or verbally, even with a professional therapist. Talking would sometimes make me vomit, become teary with emotion and sometimes bring on chest pain from hyperventilation.

Repressing all thoughts and feelings was one reason for this. In my case art therapy was an obvious choice as words are not necessary; much can be achieved without them.

Repression, or the brain's attempt to send difficult thoughts straight into the unconscious, supported me in handling my trauma. This phenomenon is observed frequently in trauma victims who claim to have no recollections of the disturbing events. Some experts view art therapy to tap into these unconscious thoughts and memories and bring them to the surface, so that individuals can heal and reconcile them.

You're probably familiar with the left-brain and right-brain theory, which has been common knowledge among the public for quite some time now. The act of **'creative expression'** *utilizes*

the right-brain hemisphere. What's interesting is that the right brain is also where visual memories are stored. Many theorize that the two is therefore very closely linked and that this is one of the reasons that art therapy has been so successful at uncovering repressed, unconscious images.
(Theresa Burke, Ph.D.)

EMDR had made me realise that I could be expressive in my thoughts and through art, I personally was able to tell my story in a more constructive manner. Art had always been one of my interests as a child and I had dabbled through the years, using drawing and painting as a way of relaxation. But it had been an interest that had been cast aside for many years and to be frank I fully believed that I was never that good. Art took a back seat for a long time and only when I became ill and needed to network my mind into positive thoughts was the realisation that art therapy was my lifeline.

My initial art works during my ongoing visits to my psychologist were extremely dark and somewhat obscure. I would present my works to her and she would further understand where my mind set was regarding thoughts that haunted me daily. The demons that occupied my thought process became embellished on canvas and one work that stands out to this day, a work I deemed to be my last before a planned suicide attempt, highlights quite plainly how much hatred and sadness I had for myself and the world around me. I had truly had enough of life at this point and although I had been doing so well, my mind was still being tortured with dark thoughts triggered by the animation of life itself.

As you can see it depicts a contorted face of a woman crying. My interpretation of this I felt, was the pain my wife was feeling and the fact she was helpless in her plight to save me. Some other pictures painted around that time also show my inner most thoughts which could be interpreted in many ways and read differently by so many.

Over a period, I found art was a way to deal with my anxiety as to sit and paint took me to another place and I was soon able to sit for hours without a care in the world. I had noticed that my art was becoming quite eclectic and I was pretty much able to turn my hand to most things. I also found that my life in general was starting to become more focused and through art I was realising that I could heal, and I was now starting to find communication verbally less of a challenge.

My paintings were becoming less dark and certainly more colourful which I understand was a sign I was slowly getting better and a way I could personally gauge my progress mentally. It seemed my mind was responding, and brighter colours made me feel good. They made me feel happy and many a day's art allowed me to drift in to what I can only explain as a different dimension. A million miles away from PTSD.

As my illness continued, my hunger for art as a therapy increased. I began to utilise my skills of art by incorporating them with my love of writing. As part of my journaling, another aid to help with PTSD I decided to put a book together about my life and my experience within the ambulance service and how I had succumbed to the illness.

The cover of my book Broken designed and illustrated by myself was inspired by a vase I had seen in an antique shop.
A light bulb moment courtesy of my wife, brought the idea to life and called the book, "The broken vase" a wonderful analogy of the state I currently saw myself in. A much-loved vase that has been knocked, leaving it cracked and Broken. A vase that needed delicate repair, piece by piece. My book was eventually shortened to Broken and thanks to my wife and my continued interest in art the front cover was born.

My interest in many art forms moved me to continue writing a second book about my illness, currently in draft form, with a book cover inspired from Japanese art.

This book depicts the same jug being carried upon the back of a man standing by the shore at sunset. The jug is now complete in its form, the cracks of the jug sealed by gold and the sunset is acknowledgement that the sun is setting on a personal battle and making way for a new beginning.

The symbol of the gold sealing the cracks of the jug is symbolised in an ancient Japanese tradition, known as Kintsugi. An analogy that is now kindred with the mental struggle bestowed upon me in past years.

As a philosophy kintsugi can be seen to have similarities to the Japanese philosophy of **wabi-sabi,** *an embracing of the flawed imperfect or Japanese* **aesthetics** *values marks of wear by the use of an object. This can be seen as a rationale for keeping an object around even after it has broken and as a justification of kintsugi itself, highlighting the cracks and repairs as simply an event in the life of an object rather than allowing its service to end at the time of its damage or breakage.*

*Kintsugi can relate to the Japanese **philosophy** of "no mind" which encompasses the concepts of non-attachment, acceptance of change and fate as aspects of human life.*

"Not only is there no attempt to hide the damage, but the repair is literally illuminated... a kind of physical expression of the spirit, literally translated as "no mind," but carries connotations of fully existing within the moment, of non-attachment, amid changing conditions. ...The similarities over time, to which all humans are susceptible, could not be clearer than in the breaks, the knocks, and the shattering to which ceramic ware too is subject.

(Christy Bartlett, Flickwerk: The Aesthetics of Mended Japanese Ceramics)

I find it interesting that for hundreds of years, the Japanese were using art forms and processes within art to analogise similarities with the human mind. The use of this type of art then translates to a more physical approach to help heal the cracks in other ways such as, reiki, massage and meditation. For me, this made total sense as I personally was using these disciplines to help me through each day. This is a prime example as to how art therapy can evolve and be of benefit to an individual's wellbeing.

It wasn't long before I was using my art more to write and now illustrate children's books, something I have found a deep passion for. So ironically, there now becomes another link in that the art therapy that helped me to tell my story whilst I was struggling with PTSD…. that same principle now helps me to tell and write stories for others which I think is a fantastic outcome.

Soon I was starting to believe in myself as a person once more. My art was flowing, and people were seeing the talent and potential I had as an artist. My work soon became not just a personal thing, but I had battled to bring my work into the public domain. It was more of a self-confidence issue as still I did not feel the paintings I produced were that good. Not only did I think this, but the paintings were part of me, a private insight to me as a person and a window to my mind. Was I happy to expose that to the many?

Family and friends believed in what I was doing and felt that I should push my work for others to see. I agreed in part but furthermore on reflection felt it would once again encourage me to engage with people once more. I knew the time had come to break the shell that mental illness had enveloped me in and present the new person I had now become. To me it was like an awakening, a metamorphosis and a time to spread my wings and fly.

True enough I soon found my work adorning art galleries and art café's in far north Queensland. Commissions for my work were being requested and before long I found myself setting up a stall in Victoria. I had finally achieved the impossible. An accomplishment that took months and years to achieve. Without the belief of others, without the belief and strength in myself and without a good kick in the pants from my wife, I doubt I would have crossed the finish line and I truly doubt I would be standing here in front of you all today.

I truly believe that art therapy is a wonderful tool and should be explored as an avenue to allow PTSD suffers to gently open their minds. It is something that should be encouraged and a passion I whole heartedly believe in. The evidence is there for all to see, proof that art therapy is a viable tool to gain trust between therapist and patient and an aid to help heal. Art therapy has been used to help the military returning from combat duties. It's used in the treatment of cancer patients, children who have been exposed to traumatic upbringing, people with learning disabilities so on and so forth.

You don't have to be creative, but offer the tools to allow someone to create, to express, to heal. It is my belief that everybody has a creative side, and everyone has talent or an interest they enjoy.

The most important kind of freedom is to be who you really are. You trade in your reality for a role. You trade in your sense for an act. You give up your ability to feel and in exchange put on a mask. There can't be any large-scale revolution until there's a personal revolution, on an individual level. It's got to happen inside first.

So, to conclude I would like to leave you with this thought......

You only listen to the artist, feel the emotion, and appreciate the strength of communication within a piece of artwork created by a person with PTSD symptoms. The rediscovery of oneself, the recognition and organization of recurrent thoughts, and the ability to emote are all proven benefits that art therapy provides. Of the populations that are impacted by PTSD, of which there are many more, art therapy is a beautiful way to start a journey to coping and eventually healing. The quiet bright spaces, the pen, crayon, paper, clay, chalk, charcoal, are controlled by the person dealing with PTSD. The pace, the product, the discussion is owned by the person that feared all ownership was lost. The patience of the therapist, the recognition of ability and externalizing a problem are only a few components of this environment of therapy and these facets alone are powerful in and of themselves. If anyone could capture words swirling in the wind, (the answer as suggested by Dylan is "Blowin' in the Wind)" I would have the faith in survivors; those coping with PTSD, whose emotions captured in art forms are vibrant.

Listen to the artist!

(Art therapy.org)

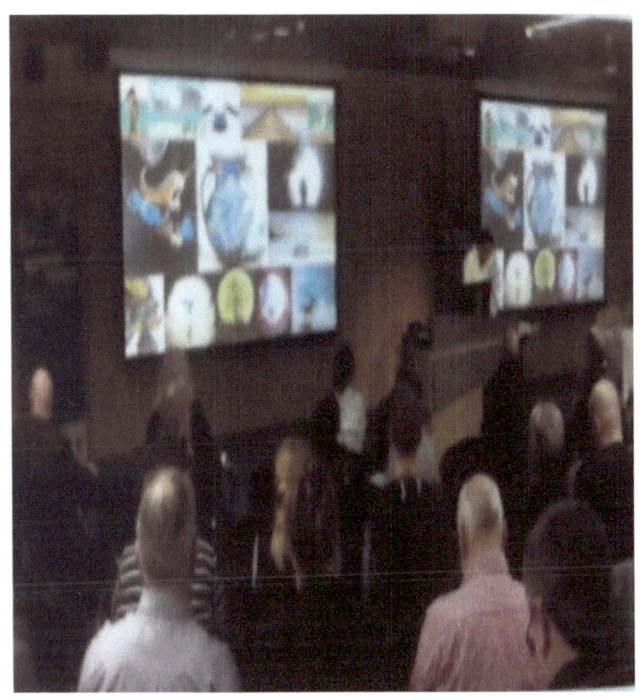

My presentation on art therapy at the paramedic symposium in Melbourne.

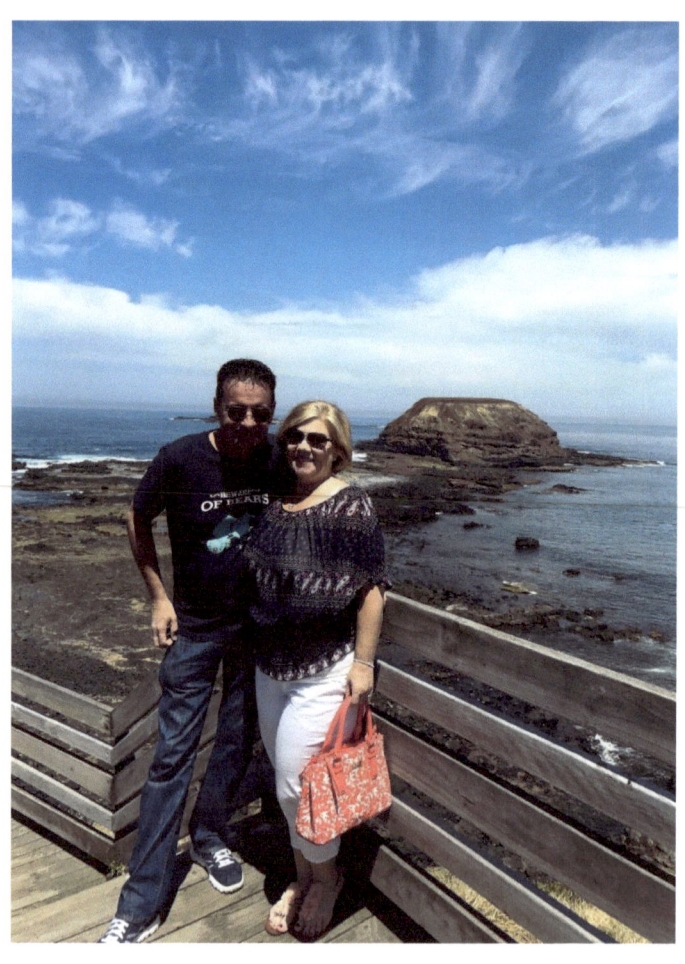

With Sharon on the Great ocean road in Victoria.

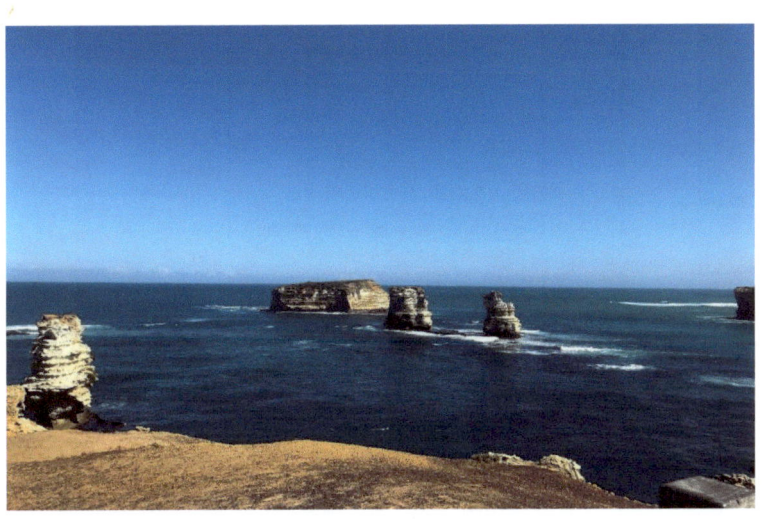

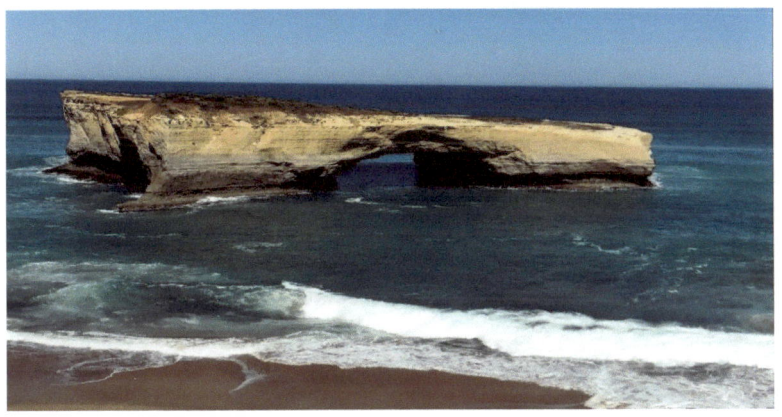

The Twelve apostles (top) and London bridge (below), Great ocean road.

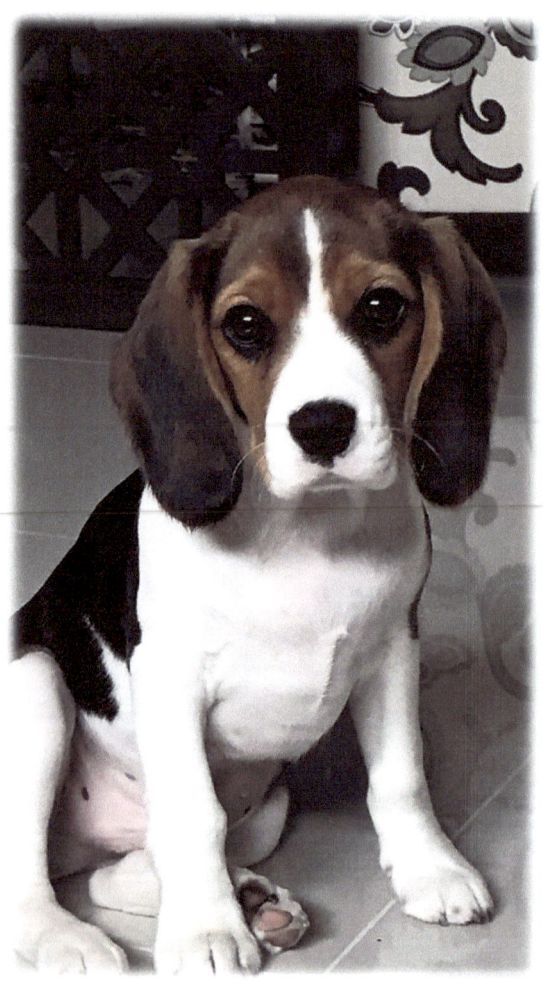

The new addition to our family – TOBY

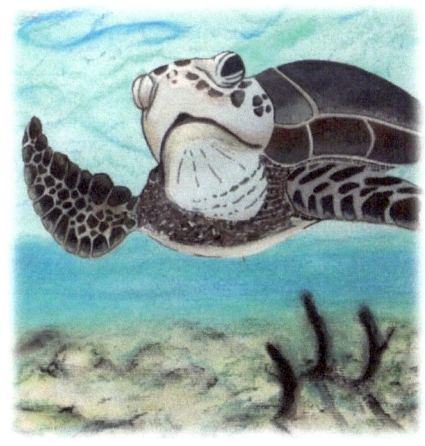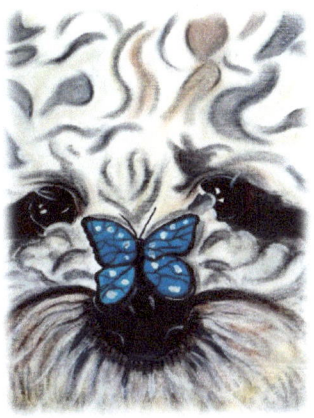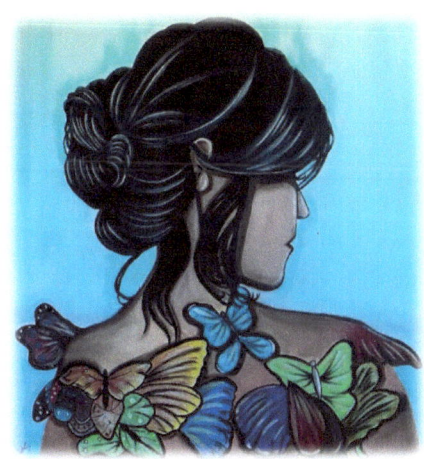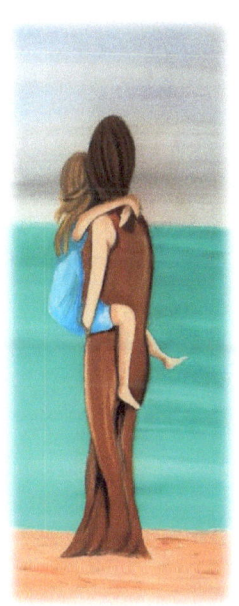

Some of my recent art work

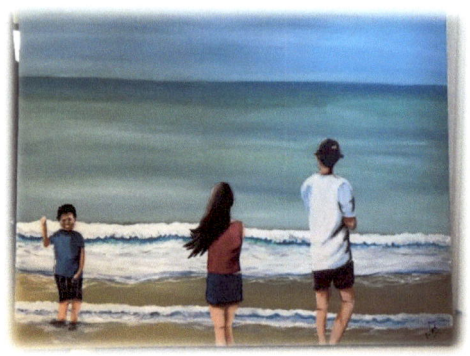
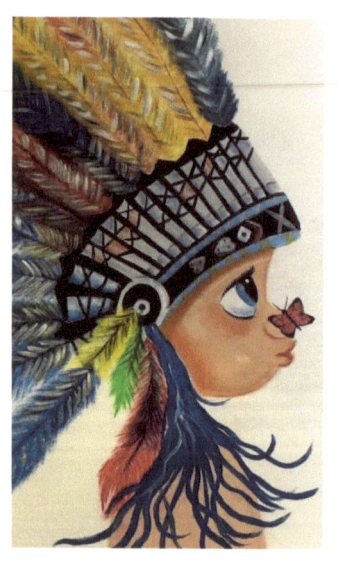
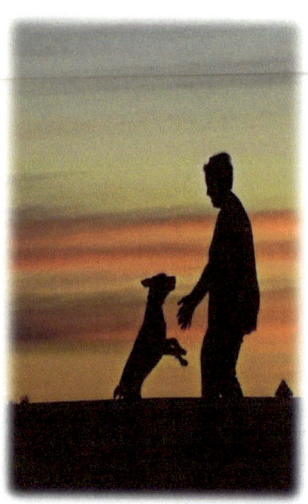

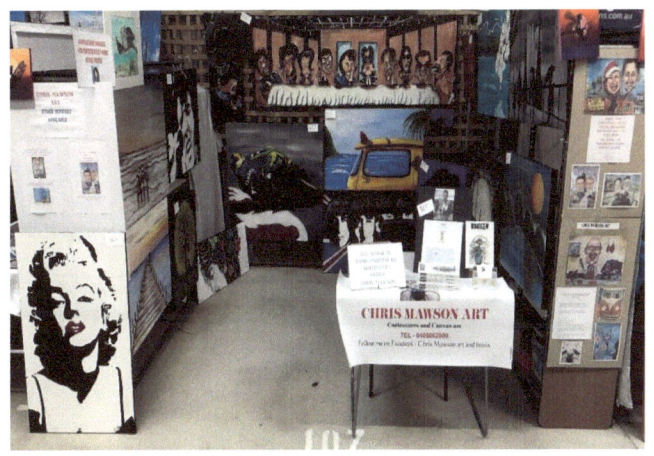

My market stall when I first started and below after expansion several months later.

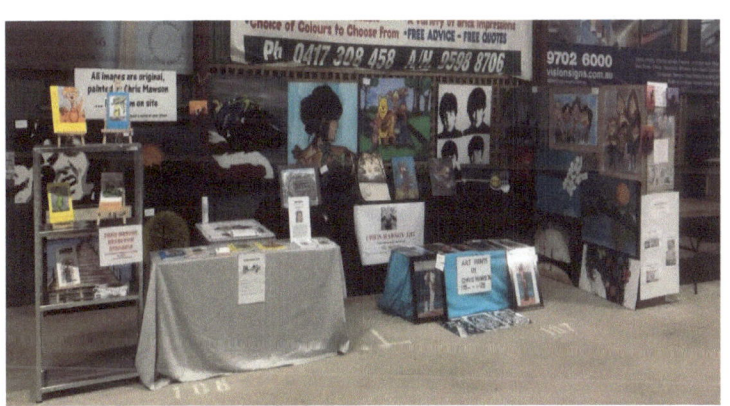

The best feeling in the entire world is watch things finally fall into place, after watching them fall apart for so long.

Patrick Ness

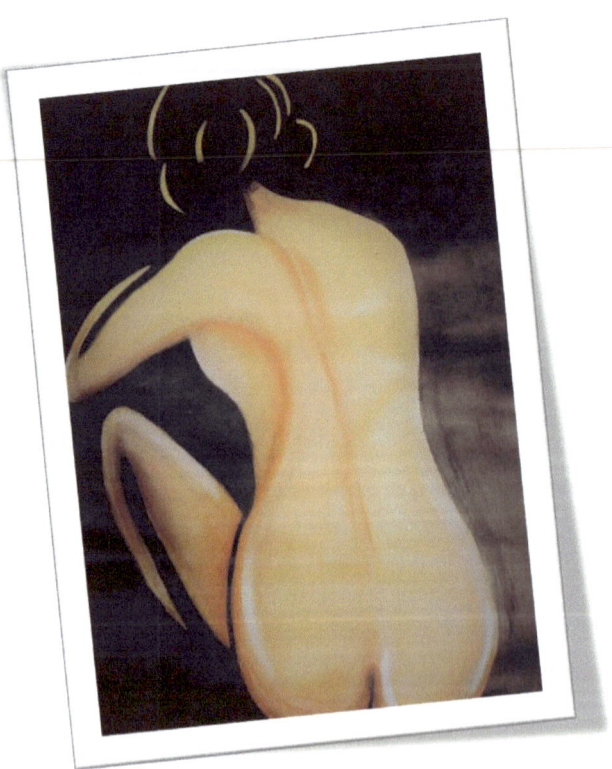

Chapter 9

AND FINALLY!!

As our life continues to flourish, doors start to open, and things start to make sense. Life up until now had been very confusing for both of us and extremely life changing. My art has taken off to a level I never expected and the belief I now have has given me the confidence to continue. The path I now travel is a good one, but it still has its bumps. I know nothing will ever be perfect, I'm not perfect. I still fight a daily battle to be who I want to be and am currently content with the person I have found within me, although I know that person is not the one I once was.

Sharon had realised that her personal goals were changing and that she had learned so much through my illness. She was a much stronger person and she was also in a better space mentally. It was time for her to follow her dreams and I was now in a better place mentally where I could support that.

My only regret is that she couldn't get the initial support she needed, whether that be from me or on a professional level. As I have said so many times before, she has been my rock and without her, I honestly don't know whether I would still be here today. The fact I am, is a true testament to a lady who has the strength of no other and it would have been so easy for her to wash her hands and walk away.

Soon after my talk at the paramedic symposium I had many contacts from people who had attended, some truly remarkable souls. They too were fighting their own battles and were all at various stages in their healing process. There is one person, who I have kept in touch with on a regular basis, his story is no different to the stories of suffering I have heard. He still fights and bears the scars, battling each day with his own demons. When I told him, I was writing this book and after his knowledge of my first book, we chatted and he told me he had been writing poems. As I have always said, creative writing, journaling or just being creative in general, is a fantastic way to open the mind and express one's feelings. Soon after our conversation I encouraged him to continue and expressed a wish to see some of the poems he had written.

His name is Russ Gregory and he sent me a fantastic piece of writing, it really sums up how important it is to understand where the true support comes from when suffering with PTSD. The wife or partner are the true hero's that live each day with the same despair, upset and sadness. For without them we are nothing.

It is my pleasure to share Russ's words -

FOREVER STUMBLING INTO HARMONY

Russ Gregory

When I become lost the absence of self-obscured reason, the foundations I had always relied on seemed to crumble beyond repair.

The rubble of these once strong beliefs left me forever stumbling. The further I stumbled the greater the disconnect from the centre became.

I knew not where to turn, many options presented but they were fleeting shadows of falsehood.

Each time I grasped and missed I spiralled further out of control, further from home.

But in the back of my mind in the core of myself was the echo of my beacon. The disarray of my spirit had masked it.

Then a soul reaches out, a small grasp of astonishing strength. The beacon of light, love and hope is a call of subliminal grounding, even during my worst loss of hope and control.

It is the call of home, the place in my heart. The constant of life in good and bad. She binds and guides me, the spirit of a dragon, the wisdom of a raven and the strength that only comes from disregard of self.

She brings me back to me, to a memory of times when life challenged us and then surrendered with the knowledge that some spirits must preserve and grow.

At the start we were separate; then two souls converged in a forest, they joined and walked a path now rarely travelled; that made all the difference.

And the reality of this joining is the truth of my life. We shine individually, but when needed we share our light; it grows from love, hope, dreams, challenge.

When we stumble we hold to each other; we are always better as one.

She is my love, my strength, my vulnerability; she is what I need when I don't know what I need.

She is my wife.

So as my story comes to an end, you may all ask, where am I now and what is in store for the future?

Well I'm still living a wonderful life in Melbourne and have no plans to move anytime soon. I am at one with my art and writing, working hard each day, but totally enjoying what I do.

Sharon now studies Naturopathy at a Melbourne university, it is her wish to one day have her own business, helping others in a more alternative way than what she is used to as a nurse. We both still have dreams, hopes and expectations. The one thing we are now grateful for is happiness.

This journey has been a roller coaster ride and it was touch and go for a while. When your life is turned upside down you have no direction, and the hand you have been dealt, is sometimes not in your favour. By staying strong, believing and getting the help you need, I promise it will set you on the healing path, just please never give up.

There are so many people I would wish to thank who without their support Sharon and I would not be the couple we are today. Naturally our families and our friends have been truly amazing in both our times of need. We are so very blessed to be part of your lives.

To my former work colleagues, you know who you all are, thank you for standing by me at the lowest ebbs of my life and I still miss you all.

To the charities that work tirelessly to make a difference and offer support for those struggling with mental illness within the emergency services, in particular- Ian and Lynn Sinclair who do an incredible job with **SIRENS OF SILENCE**. What they have achieved in the last 2-3 years is wonderful and I am grateful for the support that Sharon and I have received from them. *(To learn more about Sirens of Silence see back pages of this publication)*

Anyone else who has followed my story and picked me up along the way, thank you so very much. As I close, I shed a tear not in sadness or with heavy heart, but with the shear overwhelming love that we both feel. We are all unique in our own distinct way and life is truly a gift that needs to be cherished, 'For who knows what lies around the corner!' I deem myself to be one of the lucky ones although I know my battle continues. The path I now take is all downhill and has become easier to walk with the support and love I'm so very grateful for. All I can do now is continue to believe in all that I strive to do as an individual in life, with my beautiful wife Sharon by my side. I have so many more reasons to live than not and I'm thankful to be given that chance again.

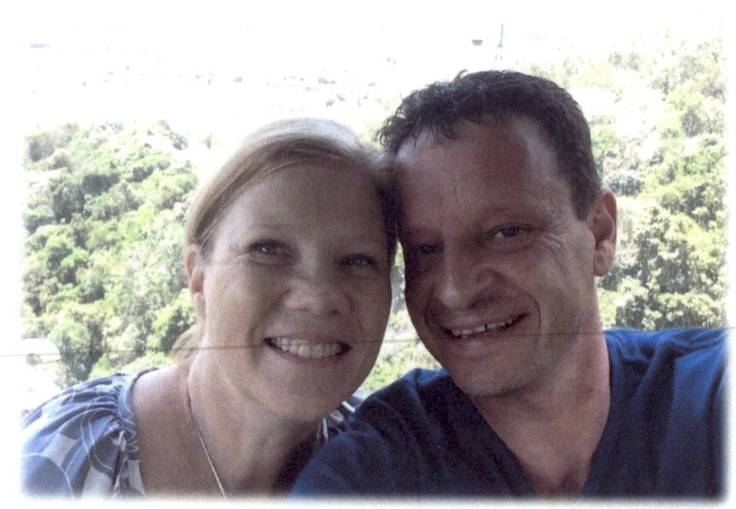

THE END

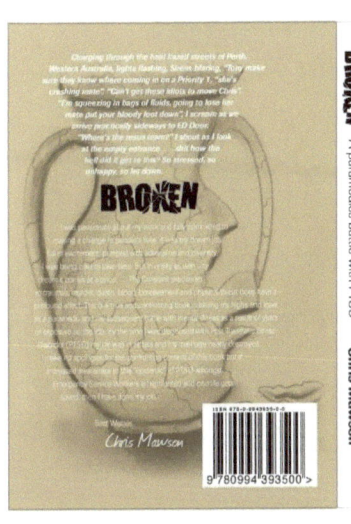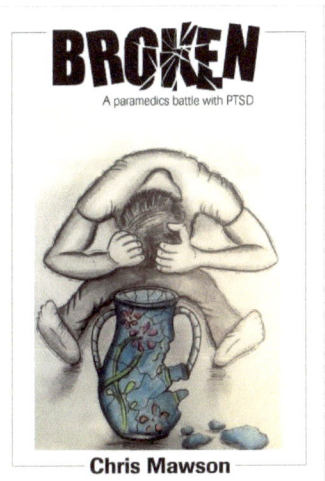

Copies of Chris's first paperback book 'BROKEN' (a paramedic's battle with PTSD), is available to purchase through Amazon.

If you wish to see more of Chris's art, you can follow him on: -

Facebook-

Chris Mawson art and books

Chris Mawson art for sale

Chris Mawson caricatures

Instagram-

Chrismawson1966

Visit him at the Akoona Market, Berwick, Victoria.

in Berwick on Sundays

CHRIS MAWSON CHILDRENS BOOKS NOW AVAILABLE THROUGH AMAZON

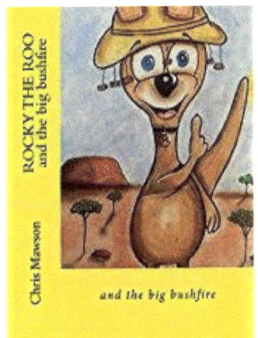
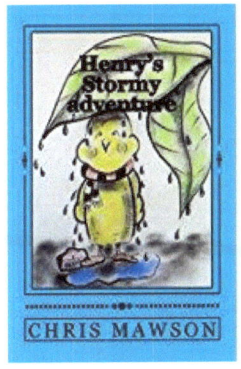
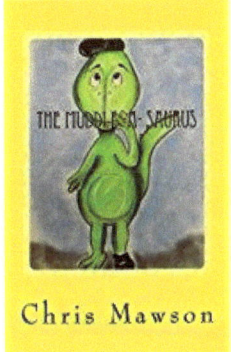
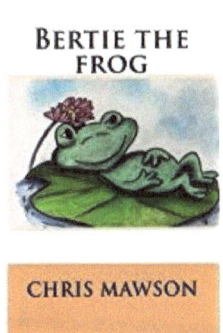
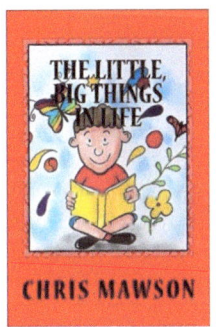

If you or a family member are struggling with any issues raised in this book and need help, please contact –

www.beyondblue.org.au

www.blackdoginstitute.org.au

www.sirensofsilence.org.au

About Sirens of silence

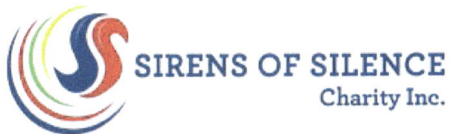

Our Principle Aim

To support all Emergency Service Personnel to engage with each other in creating a culture change to remove the social stigma that has long been associated within emergency services.

We strive to achieve a healthy future for all emergency service personnel, by providing external self help pathways and positive support to work through the difficult times.

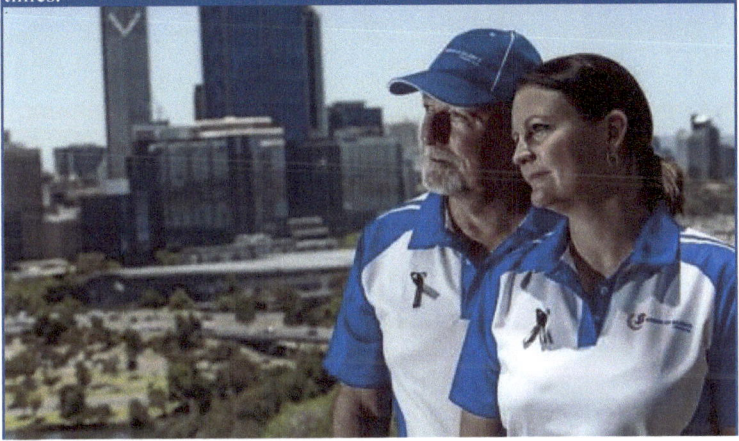

OUR STORY

Sirens of Silence Charity Inc. was founded in 2015 to raise awareness of Anxiety, Depression, PTSD and Suicide Prevention within the Ambulance Industry, it is now progressing to find supportive measures to assist ALL emergency services throughout Australia.

To take you all back to the very important beginning of our journey, 2014 was a year of shattered dreams and new beginnings not only for us, but for some of our colleagues, who we didn't realise were struggling. After I was diagnosed with a career ending injury, and having to deal with the heart-breaking decision of losing the Paramedic career I loved and worked so hard for, I struggled to find a new way forward and a new passion, whilst my husband is forever scarred by his own issues with work, he is still a passionate Paramedic in the north of W.A.

Sitting at home one Sunday night a story aired on channel 7 late in 2014 about a police officer who struggled with PTSD, which lead to his eventual suicide. His incredible story was told by his wife and aired the 000-recorded call the officer made moments before his suicide. This sad story shattered us to the core, a few weeks later a Paramedic in WA took his own life, the week after that another ambulance colleague and friend of mine took her own life. This was the 4th known ambulance personnel to suicide within 12 months in W.A. a burning pain from within lead to my new passion to help save lives and make a change into the very subject that has always been taboo for emergency services.

So, we began our new journey with a peer support page on Facebook for ambulance personnel to share stories and support each other by simply being there. Members of the page are able to share feelings and suggestions to help each other work through the emptiness. After the loss of a 6th Ambulance employee in W.A. within 14 months, we decided a serious change in culture was required from the ground up. With great support for change from those that matter on the ground, we put wheels in motion and started our National Remembrance Day for the 'In our Hearts" ribbon campaign which we launched at our first Mental Health Seminar in December 2014.

Within 4 weeks 2000 ribbons were distributed around Western Australia, Victoria, Queensland and the Northern Territory. December 22nd is our National Day of Remembrance for those we have lost. So the next step forward could only mean one thing, a charity to help those who look to be slipping through the net, so began Sirens of Silence Charity Inc.

Our principle aim is to support all emergency service personnel to engage through 'trust and honesty' about the issues that have previously been taboo, PTSD coupled with life struggles. All emergency service personnel suffer the normal stressors of life in addition to the added stressors of continual traumatic emergency service front line work. Sirens of Silence Charity Inc.

has exciting times and projects ahead, we look forward to having everyone join our team and from the ground up help make the cultural change that is long overdue.

Lyn and Ian Sinclair.

www.ingramcontent.com/pod-product-compliance
Lightning Source LLC
Chambersburg PA
CBHW040218220526
45473CB00001B/41